THE FUTURE AFTER COVID

Futurist Expectations for Changes, Challenges, and Opportunities After the COVID-19 Pandemic

JASON SCHENKER

THE FUTURE AFTER COVID

Futurist Expectations for Changes, Challenges, and Opportunities After the COVID-19 Pandemic

BY JASON SCHENKER

ISBN: 978-1-946197-48-1 *Paperback*
978-1-946197-51-1 *Ebook*

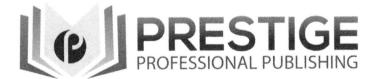

For those preparing for the future after COVID-19.

CONTENTS

CONTENTS

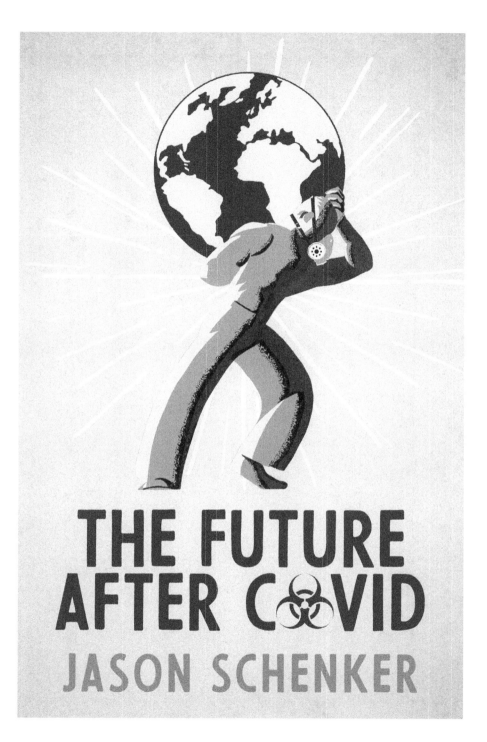

THE FUTURE
AFTER C☣VID

JASON SCHENKER

BEING A FUTURIST
IN THE TIME OF COVID-19

As a result of the COVID-19 pandemic, there have been unprecedented impacts on business, the economy, and society. But what comes next?

In *The Future After COVID*, I offer a futurist perspective.

The big idea of this book is to explore some of the most important potential long-term changes, challenges, and opportunities that the COVID-19 pandemic is likely to hold for over a dozen different critical fields and industries, including the future of work, education, healthcare, supply chain, and more.

The impact of COVID-19 is likely to cast a shadow— in both bad and good ways — across the years and decades ahead. It will impact how we work, where we live, and what different industries will look like in the future.

This book draws on research, courses, and training materials from The Futurist Institute's Certified Futurist program.

Some of the themes, topics, and content in this book draw on my other futurist books.

Changing Dynamics and Risks

This book represents an attempt to integrate the quickly changing landscape related to COVID-19 with long-term expectations and strategy. Of course, as this book was developed rapidly, some of the realities, potential future impacts, and relevance of topics may change swiftly as well.

This makes writing a book like this a bit of a risk.

But I believe it is worth it!

People need to have a futurist framework to consider the potential long-term impacts of the COVID-19 pandemic breakout, disease spread, healthcare challenges, economic fallout, work adaptations, potential impact on consumption habits, and other dynamics.

I have tried to craft this book in a way to identify trends that seem most likely to continue, change, accelerate, or end as a result of the impacts of COVID-19. But there is also a discussion of uncertainties as well.

Acknowledgements

No book is done completely alone. There are editorial, file conversion, design, and project management parts of the project to get a book like this completed. And those tasks require a team.

Along those lines, I want to thank The Futurist Institute and Prestige Professional Publishing staff for making this book a reality. And I want to especially thank **Nawfal Patel**, who managed the production of *The Future After COVID*.

I also want to thank **Kerry Ellis** for her fine work on the cover of this book. For this cover, I wanted a medical-type image of Atlas holding up the world to convey both the serious nature of the COVID-19 pandemic and how truly worldwide a tragedy and burden it is — especially for our medical and healthcare professionals. Our Atlas isn't just wearing a mask, but he also appears to be wearing scrubs, and there is a backdrop of light to convey optimism. I know it sounds like I asked a lot of Kerry — and I did. But she nailed it. I am grateful. Thank you, Kerry!

Most importantly, I want to thank my family for supporting me in my education, career, entrepreneurship, and authorship. I am always most grateful for the support of my loving wife, **Ashley Schenker**, and to my wonderful parents, **Janet and Jeffrey Schenker**. My family supports me in countless ways by providing emotional support and editorial feedback. Every time I write a book, it's a crazy experience that spills over into my family life, so to them and to everyone else who helped me in this process: Thank you!

Finally, thank you for buying this book. I hope *The Future After COVID* helps you better navigate these uncertain times!

~ Jason Schenker

CHAPTER 1

THE FUTURE AFTER COVID

The events of the past two months have felt a lot like the time just after September 11, 2001. Now — as then — people have become scared. They have become increasingly afraid to travel or go out.

And at times, it felt like the other shoe would drop.

But there are some critical and important positive differences.

Today, the economy has a greater chance to continue (at least in part), even with these disruptions. E-commerce allows people to shop and spend. This is critical because over 70 percent of the U.S. economy is driven by people buying stuff.

Many nonessential, nonremote service jobs are at risk — and they will be lost.

But more remote jobs and supply chain jobs will be created. This process has been going on for some time. Now, jobs in these areas are poised to accelerate.

Another big positive is that people can engage in remote work because of advances in business technology and innovation.

When I talk about "the future of work," I often tell clients and audiences that someday in a couple decades, I expect a child to ask me someday what work and life were like back in the "old days." And when that happens, I will describe commuting to work and offices. I also expect that child will laugh at me in disbelief and say, "That makes no sense. I don't believe you."

For all of the coronavirus concerns, I am grateful that e-commerce and telecommuting exist today. And I am also hopeful that people may now be more willing to embrace online learning to find their place in the world — and improve their lot in life.

The Future After COVID affords me the chance and opportunity to share my expectations in the short run and the long term — across industries, the economy, and society.

The big takeaway that I hope this book gives you is that while there will be many significant losses and costs associated with COVID-19, there may yet be opportunities — even in these most challenging of times — to discover ways to improve public health, education, and economic outcomes in the long run.

Let the COVID-19 pandemic provide us with lessons to be learned, lest we lose the opportunity to be better prepared — and better equipped — to manage risks like these in the future. Because there will be a future after COVID-19.

CHAPTER 2

THE FUTURE IS
BEING A FUTURIST

Futurists are going to be increasingly important for helping people and organizations think about the future.

Of course, people define futurists in different ways. And there are various folks who consider themselves futurists, and they fall into a few camps.

First, there are academic futurists. They usually operate out of universities and produce academic literature. Their focus is on frameworks rather than specific problems and industries.

Second, there are people who call themselves futurists who are essentially future fanboys. Some of these people have an almost religious optimism about the future, insomuch as some of them believe that the future will always be better.

Third, there are applied futurists. This is what I do — and what The Futurist Institute trains people to do.

This is for futurists who work as analysts, consultants, or strategists. We try to create and use futurist theories — and apply them to the practical — to come up with ways to think about alternative future scenarios.

Futurists like me think about what the most important levers, drivers, and change agents of the future are. We look at what the big risks and opportunities are, and we examine what trends and underlying fundamentals might not change. Looking at change agents — as well as the big themes and trends that are unlikely to change — helps to foster and lead constructive discussions around what the future may hold.

After all, the future is not certain. But we need to think about how our expectations of the future align with fundamentals of human nature, technological development, and historical trends.

It's also important to frame discussions in terms of technologies that are likely to be broadly adopted over the coming decade — as well as those that are likely to be more important beyond that time window.

The team at The Futurist Institute and I refer to this time dichotomy as the "almost now" / "maybe someday" dynamic.

Knowing what is going to be most critical in a near-term time window is just as critical as being able to identify those that could be more important further in the future.

For example, expecting more broad-based remote work is something we have seen in the "almost now" 10-year window for the past four years. But remote working off-planet is something we continue to see as "maybe someday."

In truth, limiting the number of "maybe someday" discussion points is critical for getting corporate and organization buy-in.

The Future is for Futurists

Long-term analysts and strategic planning around trends and technology are going to become more critical going forward. For this reason, as we look ahead at the future, we expect being a futurist will become an increasingly important profession.

CHAPTER 3

THE FUTURE OF WORK

People have been able to work remotely for some time.

When I started worked in consulting at McKinsey in 2007 — almost 13 years ago — many consulting firms, including my own, were letting people work from home, and they were already using flex space and co-working spaces.

But many corporations have resisted the move to remote working environments.

In truth, when I founded Prestige Economics in 2009, it was always designed to be a remote work company. We have never had an office. And there have never been any plans to get one.

With the recent developments of COVID-19, this decision makes me feel a great deal of affinity for the motto, "I'd rather be lucky than good." Although pandemic risks have always loomed out there, the fact that we are now living through one of this magnitude has proven to be an unexpected surprise for many.

We are now at a watershed moment. And while the ability to have large remote working staff has been a potential for many years, companies that resisted the move are now being forced to adapt.

Going forward, many companies will likely be unable to wind the clock backward.

Of course, some companies will never look back. They may continue to support remote work, which reduces corporate overhead and increases worker satisfaction and flexibility.

Other companies may wish to reverse the trend. But now that people are working remotely — and many of them very effectively — companies that wish to reverse the trend and end remote working conditions are likely to find it difficult to get their workers back in the office full time.

Three Kinds of Jobs
Beyond the changes in remote work, there has also been a new realization about three kinds of jobs — three kinds of workers:
> — **Essential Workers**
> — **Knowledge Workers**
> — **Everybody Else**

First, there are essential jobs for essential workers. These are jobs people have to show up for. Essential jobs are in healthcare, utilities, manufacturing, agriculture, supply chain, and other critical industries that keep the economy going — and contribute to societal stability overall.

The second category of workers are knowledge workers. They have jobs that can be done remotely. This includes entire industries, like many jobs in technology, finance, and many other fields. In addition to entire professional fields that can operate remotely, some office, administrative, and executive staff at essential companies can also work remotely.

Finally, there is a third category of jobs.

It's essentially everything else. Unfortunately, there are a lot of people in those jobs that can't work remotely — and jobs that are not considered essential.

These are a lot of service-based jobs, and these include people who work in restaurants and bars, movie theaters and casinos, hair salons, and nail salons. In total, there are lots and lots of jobs that fall into the nonessential, nonremote bucket.

In 2001, during the recession, I ended up waiting tables. It was a job that required minimal training, and if you worked hard at it, you could earn a decent income to sustain your existence. But now, in an era of the COVID-19 pandemic, waiting tables is not an option.

I wonder what I would do today as a future or recent graduate, entering a job market with COVID-19-induced hiring freezes in place and having only a relatively limited network, work experience, or professional skills.

Perhaps I would be working for Instacart or Uber Eats.

Healthcare Jobs

As a result of experiencing the COVID-19 pandemic, it seems likely that people may consider going into healthcare fields. And I expect there will be a few reasons for this. For some people, it will likely be a mix of these.

First, I expect that there will be an increased preference to prepare for careers as healthcare professions from students in universities and colleges. Some of these people may change their majors as they see some of their peers experience the negative job market impacts of a COVID-19-induced recession. As other potential professional options dwindle, some students are likely to seek out healthcare to be recession-proof. After all, healthcare is certainly a field well known for that.

In fact, the recession-proof nature of healthcare is something I have discussed in several of my books, including *Robot-Proof Yourself*, *Jobs for Robots*, and *Recession-Proof*.

Second, I expect that we will see increased interest in the medical and healthcare professions from midcareer professionals who lose their jobs, are at risk of losing their jobs, or who seek to retool and reskill in order to have more job security in the long run.

Healthcare workers are in high demand, and healthcare job categories have long been recognized by the U.S. Bureau of Labor Statistics as critical growth areas in the decade ahead. An aging population, increased longevity, and rising national wealth are all likely to contribute to increased healthcare needs in the future.

Third, I expect that we will see an increased preference to be in healthcare from people who are not yet in postsecondary schools. Some of these pupils may choose this profession as a way to contribute to the struggle against pandemics and help improve public health.

In the same way that some people enlisted in the military after the attack on September 11, 2001, we may see people choosing to go into healthcare as a calling — as their patriotic duties.

Again, some people may get into healthcare for a wide variety of reasons — to improve their job chances in the immediate term, to improve their long-term prospects, or to answer a calling.

But no matter what the reason is behind people's decisions to go into healthcare, it is a profession and a field that is likely to remain evergreen in a world of economic uncertainty, financial market volatility, pandemic risks, and automation. It is also a field that is not funded by discretionary income.

After all, if you need medical treatment, you need medical treatment. It's not like the tourism industry, which can see wild volatility around GDP and equity markets.

Healthcare is a constant that people will continue to need, regardless of the economy.

Careers in healthcare are also likely to be solid for a long time to come, since the demographics of an aging U.S. population will necessitate expanding the ranks of frontline healthcare professionals, including personal care aides, registered nurses, and home health aides. In *Jobs for Robots*, I presented information about the positive outlook for healthcare job growth, and in the table below, Figure 3-1, you can see the current expectations for job growth by occupation in the U.S. economy.

Healthcare is the clear winner.

Additionally, when we think about the potential to automate, it is important to recognize that not all jobs are easy to automate.

Figure 3-1: Greatest Number of New Jobs by Occupation[1]

Most New Jobs: 2018-2028

OCCUPATION	NUMBER OF NEW JOBS (PROJECTED), 2018-28
Personal Care Aides	881,000
Food Preparation/Service Workers	640,100
Registered Nurses	371,500
Home Health Aides	304,800
Cooks, Restaurants	299,000
Software Developers	241,500
Waiters and Waitresses	170,200
General and Operations Managers	165,000
Janitors and Cleaners	159,800
Medical Assitants	154,900

Source: Bureau of Labor Statistics

FI   THE FUTURIST INSTITUTE

And healthcare jobs, especially those with high levels of human contact, are likely to be resilient, even in the face of greater levels of automation across the broader economy.

This should not be a small consideration when thinking about jobs in the long run. After all, in the future, many jobs will cease to exist because of automation. This is something driving the U.S. Bureau of Labor Statistics' forecasts for job creation and losses by profession shown in Figure 3-2.

As we look at the categories with the greatest growth potential, we again see healthcare is the top winner. It's a need not a want, it's not easy to automate, and demographics favor the healthcare field. It is the definition of essential. What more do I need to say?

Figure 3-2: Healthcare Job Creation Tops the List[2]

Fastest Growing Jobs: 2018-2028

OCCUPATION	GROWTH RATE, 2018-28
Solar Photovoltaic Installers	63%
Wind Turbine Service Technicians	57%
Home Health Aides	37%
Personal Care Aids	36%
Occupational Therapy Assistants	33%
Information Security Analysts	32%
Physicians Assistants	31%
Statisticians	31%
Nurse Practitioners	28%

Source: Bureau of Labor Statistics

FI   THE FUTURIST INSTITUTE

Change is the Only Constant

The U.S. labor market is always changing. You can see that in Figure 3-3. In the mid-1800s, the majority of the workforce was agricultural. Today, agricultural jobs comprise less than 1 percent of the entire U.S. labor force.

But there have been other big changes as well. Manufacturing peaked in the 1970s but has since fallen, while some fields, like supply chain, that weren't on anyone's radar just a couple years ago have exploded. You can see the rise in supply chain jobs over the past two decades in Figure 3-4. In truth, supply chain is a field where the need for people is almost as great as the need for automation.

Figure 3-3: The U.S. Labor Market[3]

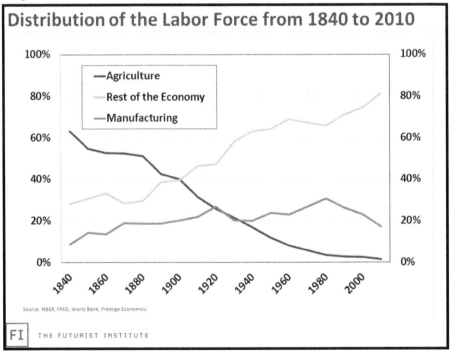

After all, the COVID-19 pandemic response revealed that there is a greater need for automation, AI, and robots — especially in the supply chain. Technology in our supply chain has been stressed to the limits of its capabilities, as it has been deployed as the lifeline of the economy to meet consumer demands, despite very thin inventories that are broadly disbursed.

The COVID-19 pandemic has forced us to cross a critical threshold for e-commerce. Now, it is no longer just a convenience; it is a pure necessity. And that will be even truer in the future. Automation will be critical, because people alone could not do everything necessary to meet the economic needs of the supply chain. But looking ahead, I still expect more people will be working in supply chain in the decade to come.

Figure 3-4: Supply Chain Jobs[4]

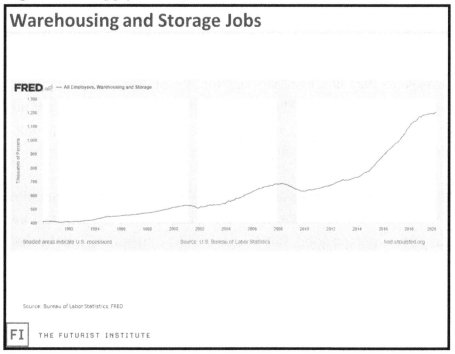

Knowledge Workers and Remote Work

Beyond healthcare and supply chain, there are also big value propositions for seeking out jobs with a high technology component — jobs that can be done remotely. This is something many people have been working on for some time, but now COVID-19 has again revealed a critical open secret: Being able to work remotely using technology and being a knowledge worker, can keep your job alive — even in disruptive time.

The value adds for remote work jobs are clear. For workers, telecommuting saves time, fuel, and other costs. Meanwhile, for employers, there's a cost savings from a reduced need for commercial office space, parking spaces, equipment, and office supplies. Reliability is also arguably higher when people telecommute, even if there are additional cybersecurity risks as corporate attack surfaces and knowledge infrastructure become more distributed.

Everyone that has ever worked for me at Prestige Economics, which I founded in 2009, has telecommuted. We don't have an office because we don't need one. All I care about is that people complete their tasks completely, correctly, and on time.

If we look at the professional jobs of the future, they are remote. Healthcare, supply chain, manufacturing, and trades will still be largely in-person jobs. But business jobs and professional roles will be mostly online. This is something that has been brewing for some time. And the increased societal and economic preferences for healthcare jobs, supply chain jobs, and remote jobs could very well be permanent, long after the COVID-19 pandemic has ended.

CHAPTER 4

THE FUTURE OF EDUCATION

The future of education is online.

I've had this expectation in the past, and it's one that I have professionally embraced and continue to hold.

In my 2017 book *Jobs for Robots*, I discussed how online education has a chance to significantly better society — and how education is the greatest tool humans have to stay relevant in a world of increased automation.

The Trend is Your Friend

The rising trend in online education has been gathering steam for some time, and now we are seeing that COVID-19 has forced essentially all learners out of classrooms and online.

This is happening at all levels of education — primary, secondary, postsecondary, professional, certificate, and informal.

Of course, there's also been significant growth in online courses on platforms like LinkedIn learning. And the general trends in massive online open courses (MOOCs) and simultaneous massive online courses (SMOCs) have been growing for a long time. But, of course, this hasn't just been a growth in informal education.

In truth, all of these courses are likely to grow.

Trends tend to build slowly and then accelerate at certain threshold moments. This may be that moment for online education. And the current experience alone may be enough to change the future of higher education as well as all forms of education permanently.

I've shared the story in other books about how I completed my third full master's degree entirely online without ever going to a campus. This included defending my master's project remotely, as well as doing teamwork and group projects online.

And I was doing that back from 2014 to 2016.

Of course, the technology is even better now.

The tools people have are better now. Computers are faster now; smartphones are better now. Essentially, everything people need to be their most successful with online learning has all improved drastically in the years since I completed an entire master's degree online.

And as I look to the future of education, I see the potential for three main dynamics to come out of the COVID-19 pandemic experience.

These are the same three dynamics that have affected other industries where technology helps to break a guild system and education is — especially at the collegiate and post-collegiate levels — a guild system.

That's what the entire model of doing a bachelor's degree, master's degree, and Ph.D. is based on; it's based on the medieval structure of apprentice, journeyman, master.

Those three levels roughly are equivalent to what one would have seen in either knighthood or in medieval formal degrees. The Ph.D., the doctoral degree, is the pinnacle of these, and a dissertation was designed to roughly mirror the *Meisterstück* or *chef d'oeuvre* — the masterpiece — which would make one a *Meister* — a master of their field. Although the words we use in education are different, the structure of higher education is still medieval in nature.

Historically, that guild structure has often been a barrier to entry for many careers and disciplines. But online education has tremendous potential to disrupt traditional studies and the guild of the academy by drastically expanding the reach of course materials and education content. I expect this is what we're going to see at an accelerated pace in the years to come. More people will be educated than ever before online — and in total, because of online education.

Three Trends in Education

The three trends that we've seen in FinTech — cost disintermediation, democratization, and improved user experience — are the same three drivers I expect will impact the future of education.

First, is the ability to disintermediate education costs by breaking the education guild system. Second, is the ability to democratize access with an online platform and educate more people. And third, there is the chance to improve the learning experience.

Even though most people might think of college or grad school as a time to be in an archetypical suburban or even rural campus environment where lots of the learning process is organically supported by the life experience of being in a certain kind of conducive environment, that's about to change in a big way.

In recent years, smaller colleges have come under financial pressure. Now, with both an economic slowdown and increased move to online education, I expect that we are going to see some small colleges come under enough financial pressures in the near term to shutter their doors.

And while some small liberal arts colleges — or colleges that resist an expansion online — may cease to exist, large universities are likely to see this as a tremendous opportunity to help fulfill and expand their mandate. After all, they will be able to serve many, many more people by increasing access to online education. And they may be able to do so at a price point that more people could afford.

It's important to remember that most people get into education because they want to help people learn. This is true in primary, secondary, postsecondary, and professional education.

The ability to help more people is something that educators would likely see as a greater calling than serving fewer people, provided that the learning actually happens. There is this really critical concern that if you expand the number of learners, that you may actually decrease the quality of the education.

However, the online education experience of the COVID-19 pandemic response is likely to demonstrate that it is possible to provide effective, quality education even while drastically increasing the numbers of students. If this proves true, which I expect it generally will, the biggest and most well-known universities could push to drastically increase the number of students they serve online, which could disintermediate cost.

Education Inflation Outstrips Total Inflation
Education costs have greatly outstripped other costs. You can see this dynamic when examining the education subindex of the U.S. consumer price index (CPI) inflation data when compared to the total CPI.[1]

In Figure 4-1, you'll note that the education costs have almost always outstripped average year-on-year growth rate in total inflation. Needless to say, uninterrupted, this trend is likely to prove unsustainable for the future of education affordability and access. And it's one of the main reasons why online education is likely to explode in terms of adoption.

The ability to serve more people at a low price point and create competition could break the higher education guild and disintermediate cost, providing a massive societal benefit where more people would be able to get more significant education on demand. In *Jobs for Robots*, I wrote about online education as the in-hand classroom, and indeed this is something that has been a potential for some time. Now, we appear likely to see a leap above the previous threshold.

It's also the reason I founded The Futurist Institute back in 2016. And it's why our courses have always been online. We wanted to be able to serve the maximum number of learners possible at a low price point.

Figure 4-1: Education CPI[2]

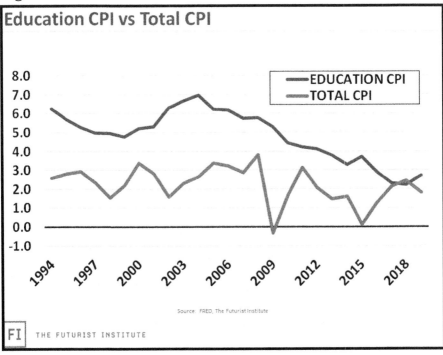

This is how business works, and even though universities are often not-for-profit institutions, they, too, are still businesses of sorts. After all, university budgets must balance and they also have a mission. But rather than focusing on profits, the mission is to effectively educate as many people as possible.

This is a critical piece, especially when we think about the future of work and we look at the education threshold as being a critical precondition for success as a telecommuter or as a remote worker. In other words, you must be a knowledge worker, and you really need to have a high level of skills or education in order to effectively work online in many cases.

After the COVID-19 pandemic these two dynamics will fold together, where the desire for education will greatly increase because those are the jobs that are pandemic proof. And those will be the jobs that people will want in ever increasing numbers, which means that demand for education will rise since both aspiring knowledge workers and universities will have been forced to cross the Rubicon of online education.

They will likely be able to find ways to continue to serve more people and to more effectively fulfill a broadened scope of their mission to educate people while also increasing the efficacy with which a larger number of people could be educated, at least at a greater way than ever before.

Beyond the disintermediation of cost and this democratization of access, there is also the improved user experience. And this is where we see the technology being a lever.

Paying Elite Tuition Without In-Person Benefits

One of the reasons we may also see a disintermediation of cost in education is because parents who are paying college tuition — or students who are paying their own tuition — to universities to the tune of tens of thousands of dollars per semester, may realize that they can get the same amount of education remotely, just by watching it online.

This realization may push some students and their parents to seek out alternatives in order to get through their courses more quickly, or they may decide that the education value isn't really why they're at the most elite universities.

One of the biggest arguments in favor of elite education is that it introduces you to a network. But that network is a lot more distant when it's remote. And really elite institutions of higher education have been offering online courses for some time.

Harvard has offered courses through its extension school since 1910. And it has been offering online courses and degrees for a number of years at a fraction of the cost of the traditional courses at Harvard University. Of course, there is a distinction between being at Harvard University versus the extension school. But it's probably not that big to most people. After all, it's still Harvard.

And Harvard isn't the only school that offers online courses, remote courses, online certificates, and other programs. Many universities do this. I've personally done certificates online with MIT and Carnegie Mellon. If the content is your priority, then for some learners, the online experience may be most effective.

Of course, online courses force you to miss out on some of the biggest potential of going to an elite institution: networking.

Whether we are talking about online courses, remote courses, or hybrid courses, I expect that the future of education following the COVID-19 pandemic is likely to lead to two critical outcomes.

In addition to expecting an increase in total education attainment at the population level following the COVID-19 pandemic, I also expect an acceleration in the number of explicitly designed online courses. And I believe there could be pushback against some advanced education with very high costs.

After all, people have been more willing to accept the high cost of education in the past, because it came with a guaranteed network. But it's very tough to build long-term relationships with influential professors, thought leaders, Noble laureates, and your academic peers, who may someday be future leaders, if you are only taking a course online that was envisioned, designed, and sold as an in-person value add. The truth is that if the networking is the real value-add (which seems to be the case) and the education is secondary, then the cost of elite university education as well as elite liberal arts college education might suffer some pushback on price, and there could be a preference for networking experience outside of the academy as a substitution effect for the lost networking value.

This isn't a guarantee, of course, but this is just one potential side effect we could see from people watching their children take $20,000 or $30,000 worth of courses online like they're just watching YouTube videos.

The Value Add of Technology

Technological aids are likely to decrease the cost of education and increase the potential for competition. And we also see a significant potential for technology to support democratized access to education and improve the learner experience.

Furthermore, the use of technological aids will only likely improve over time. And if we see universities remain closed for the spring semester of 2020, technological aids that improve the online education user experience could become more critical. At the time this book was published, there was a not small potential for some universities to remain closed through the end of the entire calendar year of 2020, thus canceling any summer or fall semesters for in-person courses.

To support this endeavor, I expect that we are likely to see increased investment in EdTech (education technology) as well as significant investments across tools, training materials, and remote materials that allow for a more cohesive learning process. Once we see students and teachers become accustomed to the online education delivery model using these technologies, we are likely to find people will be more accepting of them.

There's an old German saying, "Was der Bauer nicht kennt, frisst er nicht." It translates roughly as "What the farmer doesn't recognize, he won't feed on." Because guild industries like healthcare and education are based on centuries of tradition, the actual process of getting into their guilds is not necessarily steeped in technology, even in those fields themselves that are immersed in technology and embrace technology.

I expect that we are likely to potentially see some changes stemming from technological disruption to these guilds in the decade ahead — and beyond. The unique situation of COVID-19 may even hasten the process, as it has revealed a shortage of healthcare workers, while also bringing to light the tremendous potential for online education and remote work.

There are also likely to be important regional opportunities, In the state of Texas, where, I live there is an initiative known as 60 by 30; the goal is to have 60 percent of Texans age 25 to 34 complete some level of postsecondary education, degree, or certificate by the year 2030. It is an ambitious goal, but it is critical because the jobs that are remote and less automatable are critical for the next economic phase of growth in Texas. And it is exactly this cohort of jobs that requires education and technological skills.

Trade skills, formal education, informal education, and perpetual learning are all likely to gain a boost from online education. And the rise in online education due to the U.S. COVID-19 response makes Texas much more likely to achieve the 60 by 30 goal.

This is not to say that the pandemic of COVID-19 is positive. It is most certainly not. It is horrific. It is a catastrophe.

Yet, if we were to consider the impacts for the economy and society at the population level, we might say (in an attempt to find kernels of hope in a desperate situation) that now maybe in the long run our populace will be more educated — and we will have a much better prepared workforce for the decades ahead.

From an economic standpoint, this is invaluable. From a population stability standpoint, this is invaluable. And from a public health perspective, where we see there is a massive deficit of people in healthcare fields — and a massive need going forward to fill healthcare jobs — we also expect that online education will help to facilitate filling those roles in the healthcare fields going forward. If that is a result, then public health outcomes in the long run could be greatly improved.

This is a topic for discussion in the chapters about "The Future of Healthcare" as well as "The Future of Work." But it's really important as we think about the future of education to bridge that gap between the needs of the economy, the needs of the workforce, the needs of the people and public health needs, and the educational capabilities to have the workforce cross a divide that up until now seemed honestly almost insurmountable and quite daunting.

I am much more optimistic now that we will achieve improved levels of public health over time because we may be able to create not only a more educated workforce, but we are also likely to see the education enrollment in health sciences and life sciences increase in a way that may also result in a long-term positive net benefit for public health and the economy.

Again, this is not to say that COVID-19 is in any way a positive. But if we were to look at long-term ramifications, there is reason for hope that out of this pandemic tragedy and economic crisis, we might be able to derive something of value and something positive in the long run.

The Impact on Home Schooling

One dynamic that has yet to be determined is what the experience of involuntary at-home, in-hand learning will be on homeschooling.

In Figure 4-2, you can see the trend in home schooling since 1999. Both the absolute level and the percent of U.S. pupils aged 5 to 17 who are home-schooled appear to have peaked in 2012 before slowing in 2016.[3]

It seems quite likely that the COVID-induced widespread mandate for home schooling might result in an increase in home schooling in the United States. After all, the new experience for many may actually result in better outcomes for some learners.

Figure 4-2: Education CPI[4]

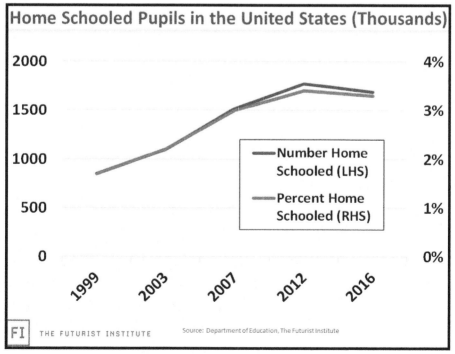

Home Schooled Pupils in the United States (Thousands)

THE FUTURIST INSTITUTE

Source: Department of Education, The Futurist Institute

Although it is not guaranteed that the number of home-schooled students will rise in the wake of COVID-19, it does seem quite likely. After all, some learners and parents may find the new experience to be preferable.

Plus, this kind of event highlights the risk to families that rely on a system outside of their control to provide for, assure of, and essentially guarantee education outcomes. Some people who planned their lives around school being an assured, undisruptable institution may demonstrate a preference for more control over such risks in the future.

Meanwhile, pupils who are home-schooled are unlikely to turn away from home schooling as a result of COVID-19. In essence, their educations and learning lives are likely to be much less disrupted than pupils in public, private, charter, religious, and other physical schools. I mean, why would they want to stop doing the only thing that works?

That seems like a less likely outcome than expecting that those now operating in a broken system of physical places of learning may cross the Rubicon of home schooling — never to return to physical buildings.

In sum, many changes are coming.

And more remote learning and at-home, in-hand education is likely to be seen across all learning levels, from home-schooled primary school pupils to undergraduate college students and doctoral candidates.

In the long run, increased access to all levels of education is likely to result in improved economic outcomes at the population level.

Historically speaking, education has been the great divider for jobs. In Figure 4-3, you can see statistics on unemployment and earnings from 2018 from the U.S. Bureau of Labor Statistics. Education is positively correlated with income, and education is also inversely correlated with unemployment. In other words, generally speaking, the more education you have, the more money you make and the lower the chance you are unemployed.

And a more educated population will be both wealthier and more employable.

Figure 4-3: Education, Earnings, and Unemployment[5]

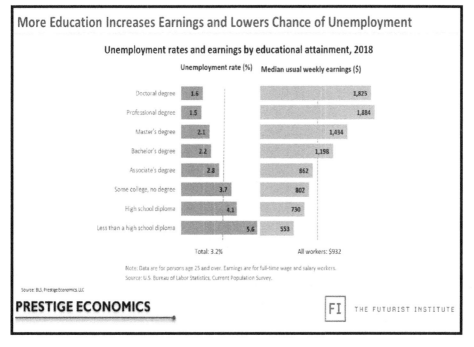

CHAPTER 5

THE FUTURE OF ENERGY

When people debate the future of energy, electric vehicles is a hot topic — and it's bearish for crude oil demand. But it ignores one much more critical factor: Global wealth is rising, and petroleum-fueled vehicles are going to become more important with the expansion of emerging market middle classes.

This means that the locus of critical oil demand is also going to shift from the OECD to the Far East and other emerging markets.

In the same way that U.S. shale oil production presents a dynamic shift in terms of the geographic source of additional marginal barrels of crude oil, the rise of the middle class in emerging markets presents a similar risk for the future of marginal additional oil demand. So, while the 2020s are likely to be a decade in which U.S. crude oil production and refineries play an increasing role in the global supply chain of crude oil, it is also likely to be a decade in which Chinese, Indian, and other Asian demand rises drastically.

COVID-19 Impacts and Telecommuting

The COVID-19 pandemic changes a few things in the outlook — especially more downside risk in the immediate term as well as the potential for some reduced upward price pressure in the medium term. But the biggest dynamics decades into the future will be the significant increases in global population and wealth. Those realities will not change.

Since the beginning of 2020, there have been three $10-ish big drops in WTI Crude Oil Prices. The first price drop coincided with the COVID-19 slowdown in China and global manufacturing. The second price drop coincided with a breakdown of OPEC+ negotiations to constrict supply, and the Saudi response to increase production. And the third price drop coincided with overall bearish market sentiment about COVID-19 negative economic impacts globally.

In the short term, COVID-19 "shelter in place" rules are de facto mandated demand destruction for transportation fuels of various kinds — especially gasoline and jet fuel.

Plus, U.S. oil production has been high. And during a shutdown period, demand destruction could push inventories to record levels in the United States, introducing both national and regional supply gluts for crude and products that are unable to move. This means that even in a post-pandemic recovery, petroleum fuels demand may remain soft, keeping prices under pressure. This could prove especially true, as more people continue working remotely against the backdrop of a potentially uncertain OPEC+ relationship between Russia and Saudi Arabia.

From a futurist perspective, however, remote work is likely to be absolutely critical for energy prices in the medium term. After all, if more people continue to work remotely, that could mitigate some of the upward pressures on rising global oil demand and prices. It is something I have expected for some time. In fact, about a decade ago, I gave a television interview to CNBC as part of a series created by Carl Quintanilla titled *Beyond the Barrel*. Although I found it personally memorable for the fact that I was wearing a white linen suit on a beach in Cancun at a meeting of the International Energy Forum, that wasn't actually the most important part of the interview.

My interview focused on the biggest potential long-term downside risk to oil prices. And although people often see and discuss electric vehicles as the main source of oil demand abatement, the main points of my interview were focused on one critical point: that telecommuting, what we are now more simply calling remote work, presents downside risk to oil demand growth — and potentially to oil prices.

From an energy standpoint, if you don't have to leave your home to go to work, you don't need to drive and you don't need to have two spaces — your home and your office — cooled or heated to account for climate control.

As you can see in Figure 5-1, telecommuting as a means of getting to work increased the most between 2005 and 2015. This growth in the telecommuting sector was already emerging in the mid-2000s, and it is a subject I discussed in my book *Jobs for Robots*.

The value propositions for increased telecommuting — or remote work, in 2020 parlance — are simple. Aside from saving time for workers, it also reduces costs for employers. Employers do not need to spend as much on commercial office space, utilities, paper products, or parking spaces if workers never come into an office. While e-commerce presents upside demand for energy in the decade ahead, the trend of telecommuting presents the opportunity to limits increases in future fuel demand.

More people are likely to telecommute over time. In fact, there could be a sustained post-pandemic bump in telecommuting. After all, the COVID-19 pandemic response has raised awareness about both remote work and online education.

Figure 5-1: The Rise of Telecommuting[1]

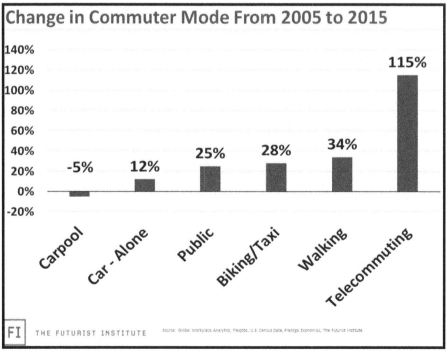

Change in Commuter Mode From 2005 to 2015

THE FUTURIST INSTITUTE   Source: Global Workplace Analytics, Flexjobs, U.S. Census Data, Prestige Economics, The Futurist Institute

Recent data reflects that telecommuters — or remote workers, as we call them today — tend to have Bachelor's degrees and graduate degrees in higher numbers than non-telecommuters. And as online education increases access to higher education, more people will have the skills to be remote workers.

Looking Ahead

Looking further out, telecommuting will continue to rise in the decade ahead. I expect this will be even more likely in developed economies, where climate change and environmental targets can be more easily met by simply lowering the number of people who drive to work or operate out of the office.

Figure 5-2: Education Levels of Telecommuters[2]

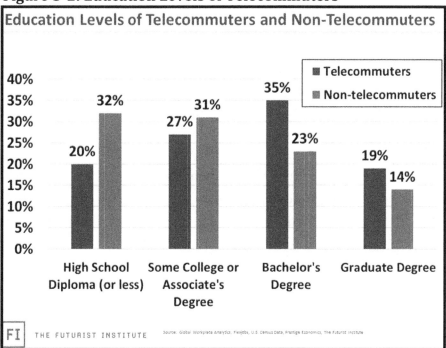

Remote work is likely to reduce petroleum fuels demand. And it is also likely to reduce power generation demand for natural gas and coal. After all, if people work from home rather than work in offices, this reduces the amount of heating, cooling, and power required in the redundant offices.

Furthermore, while renewable energy sources will be critical in the long run for power generation, natural gas offers other advantages — like not being subject to weather dynamics. At the time this book went to print, natural gas inventories were up almost 80 percent year on year. And inventories are likely to remain relatively high — even in the post-pandemic period.

Remote work seems unlikely to be a dynamic that can fully counter the future rise in energy and fuel demand over time due to significant expansions in the global population and a likely massive rise in emerging market global wealth. But telecommuting may provide some future demand abatement.

As a result of COVID-19, there has been a widespread implementation of company strategies to turn as many workers as possible into remote workers. Many of them are likely to remain remote workers. And so, you can see how the future of work, the future of education, and the future of energy come together — and could have a long-term impact on petroleum fuels and power demand.

CHAPTER 6

THE FUTURE OF FINANCE

The field of finance has been turned upside down by COVID-19.

Although individual consumers were relatively deleveraged going into this crisis, a 750 or 800 FICO credit score means very little if income ceases for weeks or months.

Plus, corporations greatly increased their leverage in recent years. This was actually the main talking point when I saw Fed Chairman Jay Powell speak at a dinner for the Atlanta Fed's Financial Markets Conference in May 2019 — almost a year ago.

Powell cautioned that business debt was high, leveraged lending was high, and CLOs were a risk.

The push to increase business leverage has been part of one of the biggest challenges of the past few years in the field of finance: the hunt for yield — the hunt for investment returns. Bond yields have been low, Treasury yields have been low, real estate prices have been up, and equity multiples have been high.

So, where were people and companies supposed to invest to generate returns?

This is a particularly gnawing question — especially if you are looking for stable fixed income investments with relatively safe returns. And this isn't just a U.S. phenomenon.

Yields have fallen almost everywhere. In Europe, the ECB still had negative deposit rates when this book went to print — and it is likely to have negative deposit rates for the foreseeable future.

These kinds of challenges could remain in play if the future of finance is one of a persistently low interest rate environment. And if central banks are going to roll out the balance sheets every time there is a downturn in the future, low interest rates could remain ubiquitous, despite activities we would have historically considered inflationary under normal circumstances.

These dynamics are also highly likely to continue into the future of finance. But that hasn't been the biggest risk in terms of chasing equity investment returns that contributed to one of the biggest losses of value in equity market history.

Unreasonable IPO Dynamics
Part of the reason equity markets took such a big a hit on concerns about the COVID-19 pandemic is because of pricing dynamics that broke from long-term equity market fundamentals. I highlighted these risks in my book *The Future of Finance is Now* (2019) and I will share them with you here.

The percentage of IPOs with negative earnings was at 81 percent in 2018 — a figure that equaled the all-time high percentage of negative earnings IPOs back in 1999, just before the tech bubble burst.[1] In 2019, that percentage fell slightly to 74 percent of IPOs with negative earnings. But that was still a very high percentage.

Historically, there has been a rising trend in IPOs with negative earnings, as you can see in Figure 6-1. But the rising trend of negative earnings IPOs during the most recent business cycle was more drastic than in previous cycles.

Problematically, this may still be common in the future, since there are now fewer public companies to invest in, and ETFs need to diversify their holdings.

Figure 6-1: Number of IPOs With Negative Earnings[2]

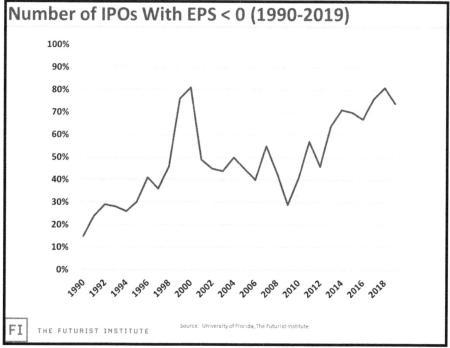

Number of IPOs With EPS < 0 (1990-2019)

But with fewer companies to invest in, that becomes a challenge for diversified equity vehicles — and it may be creating additional demand for any kind of assets available, even if they have negative earnings.

This may also partially explain why companies that have negative earnings have actually shown greater returns on their IPO days than companies with positive earnings. This dynamic can be seen in Figure 6-2. I mean, how backward is that?

Plus, the margin isn't a small one. In 2018, the average ratio of IPO-day returns for negative earnings companies was double that of companies with positive earnings. This is also true of the average IPO day returns from 1980 to 2018.[3]

Figure 6-2: Return Ratio of IPOs: Negative/Positive Earnings[4]

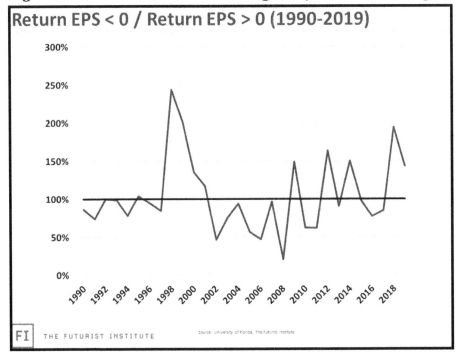

In 2019, this dynamic improved slightly, but IPO companies with negative earnings still outperformed companies with positive earnings on IPO day by almost 44 percent.

Some analysts and investors have typified this dynamic as investing in a "positive return story." In other words, people make investments because the prices have always gone up. This dynamic begins with private funding, where different rounds of funding send valuations of pre-revenue and early-stage companies ever higher. From a seed round to Series A and beyond, all the way until IPO, companies with negative earnings see their valuations rise.

We warned repeatedly in 2019 that we could continue to see the majority of IPO companies have negative earnings. The current percentage had been near historically high levels and, as I previously predicted, it "could be in for a correction in the event of a downturn."

That certainly seems likely to be the case now.

Lessons Learned and Lessons Forgotten
There's a saying among military strategists that "You prepare to fight the next war, based on the last war." And so it seems to be, too, with economists and policymakers.

We clearly forgot the frothy equity market IPO lessons of the 2000s, as we repeated them in recent years. But at least we have the mortgage and housing credit risks under control — or at least it seems we do. You know, for now.

In general, mortgage credit was shored up after the housing crisis and the Great Recession of 2007 to 2009. This is something you can see clearly in Figure 6-3, which shows new mortgage issuance by credit quality.

This data, from the Federal Reserve Bank of New York, shows a clear delineation before and after the housing crisis, where most mortgages went to people with the highest credit rating.

But even though the housing market looks secured by stronger credit, there are risks that it, too, could falter in the wake of the COVID-19 pandemic. After all, a 750 or an 800 credit score can mean nothing, if you lose almost all of your income for a month or two — or more.

Figure 6-3: Mortgage Credit Quality[5]

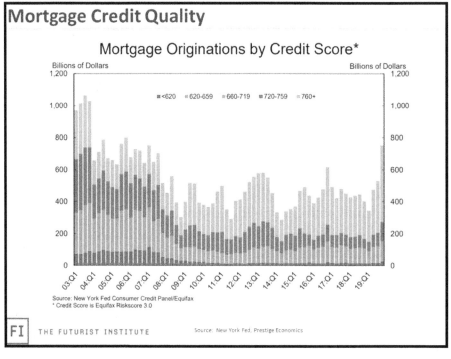

Even though the CARES act, allows for some mortgage payment deferrals and halts some evictions, this still presents a cash flow risk. And these kind of bankruptcy or eviction holidays cannot go on permanently.

At some point, these grace periods will end. And when they do, this will present downside risks to the housing market, because it could incentivize a large shock of housing supply onto the market. People who know they may no longer be able to afford their mortgages due to lost income, as well as those who are risk of permanent job loss, may try to sell their homes all at once.

This could result in a sharp increase in the supply of homes for sale at once, and it could hurt home values in the lower end of the owner-occupied housing market.

Plus, this dynamic could be particularly acute in areas where tourism is the major industry and the economic aftershocks of the COVID-19 pandemic are likely to be the most widespread. This is likely to include cities like Las Vegas, Orlando, and New Orleans. But it may also include smaller tourism and conference cities like Asheville and Austin.

This oversupply of homes nationally and regionally may happen at just the same time that demand also falls.

On the investor side, the transfer of credit risk is likely to be reflected in decreased demand for rental properties. After all, if renters can't afford their rent due to job loss, that now becomes the investor's risk.

Although the vast majority of job losses as a result of the COVID-19 pandemic are likely to be short term, it is likely that some people will lose their jobs — and most if not all of their incomes — for long periods of time. This is where the risk gets transferred from the renter to the investor owner. And if some renters just walk away from their rental agreements, this could frighten away real estate investors, further sapping housing demand, weighing on home prices.

And then there is the risk that fewer mortgages will be issued to hopeful homebuyers. In effect, the issuance of new mortgages could freeze up for a time to allow mortgage bankers and credit bureaus time to more accurately determine people's creditworthiness for the purposes of buying a home.

The impact would be reduced qualified buyers and a further reduction in home demand, further weighing on prices.

Policymakers will talk about ways to fix this, but evaluating credit is a critical risk management task of lenders. And there is only one real fix to interrupted cash flows and uncertainty of future job stability or income: time.

In sum, even though the housing credit market appears to have been shored up much more than it was before the Great Recession, there are still significant housing risks. And the end result of the COVID-19 pandemic may be that a surplus of homes hit the market as unemployment levels are elevated, and banks cannot have a clear insight into a homebuyer's credit because of interrupted income due to COVID-19.

This risk of increased owner-occupied home supply and reduced owner-occupied demand could be paired with a reduction in investor demand for rental properties, until such time as home prices fall sufficiently to offer a worthy rate of return to appropriately offset the increased risk of renter defaults and eviction risk.

Still, risks on par with the housing crisis of the Great Recession from 2007 to 2009 do not appear to be present.

Yes, there may be an increase of supply at the same time there is a concomitant drop in demand. And yes, that could weigh on housing prices — especially in high tourism areas. But it does not seem that the housing-related economic impact of COVID-19 is likely to rise to the same level of catastrophic bankruptcy and credit risk as in the last recession.

Credit Creation

In every business cycle, there is a push to expand credit, and that credit creation helps to fuel economic growth.

For most of the history of the United States, each business cycle was fueled by housing credit expansion. But that just wasn't possible after the Housing Crisis. Lending was tight. Housing credit was tight.

The result?

Credit expanded elsewhere. After all, economies always find a way to expand credit. These are the areas that present risks.

On the one hand, there was credit expansion in auto loans. And on the other hand, there was credit expansion in business credit. Let's talk about each of these.

Subprime Auto Loan Risk

The risks in housing created in the past decade pale in comparison to the credit risks associated with auto loans. As Figure 6-4 reflects, the number of auto loans in recent years has been high — with a massive surge in subprime automotive credit.

Fortunately, it is a lot easier to repossess a car than a house. But this could still present significant credit risks for banks, lending institutions, and companies specializing in automotive credit.

Figure 6-4: Auto Loan Credit Quality[6]

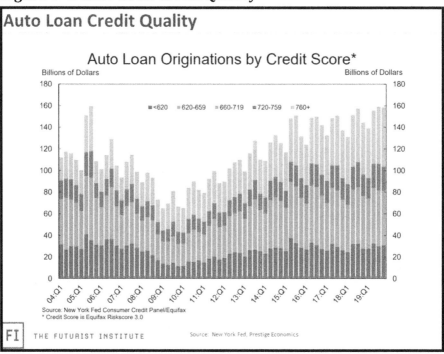

Plus, a collapse in automotive credit and a deluge of repossessed vehicles onto the used car market could hurt new auto sales. This is especially likely, if the unemployment rate remains elevated. In fact, our base case is that the unemployment rate may not fall back down to the 3.5 percent level that was seen in February 2020 — before the COVID-19 pandemic impacts — for at least two years.

This means that automotive sales could fall, and automotive credit could tighten up for years to come. Tighter automotive credit, along with tighter mortgage lending standards and a delay in new mortgage issuance, could contribute to a slow recovery. Additionally, a market flooded with auto repos could weigh on new vehicle sales. And reduced new auto sales could keep gross domestic product (GDP) growth calculations under pressure. After all, only *new vehicles* count toward GDP, which is defined as *new economic activity* in an economy during any given year.

CLOs and Corporate Debt Risks
Another major area of credit expansion in the past decade has been corporate debt. Housing credit was tight, but corporate credit had become like automotive credit in recent years: loose.

The levels of corporate debt, the amount of corporate leverage, and the proliferation of collateralized loan obligations (CLOs) introduced significant risks on the corporate side of the economic equation. The risks from these corporate debt developments to the shared national credits, credit markets, and the financial sector as a whole were the main drivers behind the U.S. Federal Reserve's March 2020 COVID-19 policy responses.

The Fed cut rates to between zero and 0.25 percent, while also massively expanding the Federal Reserve balance sheet and backing investment grade credits of various kinds — munis, asset-backed securities, commercial paper, corporate debt. Of course, lower-quality high yield credit remained exposed at the time this book was written. But the Fed could very well still jump into lower credit debt markets to save the day as well.

When thinking about the different types of economic exposures going into the COVID-19 pandemic, it's important to understand that business debt and leverage were elevated going into the COVID-19 pandemic. And although it was at record levels, this kind of debt usually rises during the business cycle.

Furthermore, this is a risk everyone knew about. It was on the Fed's radar for some time, which is why Fed Chair Powell spoke so openly about these risks at a dinner of reporters and analysts in May 2019, as I noted at the opening of this chapter.

But these business debt risks weren't a concern for investors seeking the ever-new all-time highs in equity markets, that became the bedrock of positive return stories. And the equity market story is one we have most certainly seen before — most recently in the 2001 recession.

The Next Great Credit Tightening
After the financial crisis, housing crisis, and Great Recession of 2007-2009, mortgage credit tightened up. Plus, banks and financial institutions have since had to perform various kinds of stress tests around credit and debt exposures.

Now, after the COVID-19 pandemic crisis, we could very well see a new kind of stress test — one that tests a company's ability to withstand a complete shutdown.

It seems likely that we may see increased lender requirements for companies to be able to weather two- or four-week shutdowns as a prerequisite for funding. In other words, for companies to qualify for loans in the future, they may very well need to demonstrate that they have enough cash on hand to receive funds.

As with the Coronavirus Aid, Relief, and Economic Security Act (CARES Act) bailouts, these kinds of requirements will very likely favor larger companies. Meanwhile, companies that are very small (e.g., with just a few employees) may struggle to qualify for sufficient government support to keep operations going.

Future Expectations

Looking ahead, a near-term return to equity market fundamentals seems likely. But sustained investor conservatism is too much to hope for. Additionally, there is a significant risk that fallout from the COVID-10 pandemic could have a lasting negative impact on the job market as well as the housing market.

One thing that seems uncertain in the future is if there might be a rise in inflation on the back of the CARES Act and the continued increase in the U.S. national debt. Normally, significant and sustained stimulus would engender inflationary pressures. But with the risk of a slowdown in economic growth, inflation could be staved off by deflationary risks associated with weak growth.

CHAPTER 7

THE FUTURE OF
MONETARY POLICY

One of the biggest challenges in the wake of the financial crisis was how to stimulate economic growth at a time of almost complete economic shutdown. Expanding central bank balance sheets was one of the unprecedented critical solutions that the U.S. Federal Reserve, the Bank of England, the European Central Bank, the Bank of Japan, and other central banks took to keep their economies afloat.

And as we think about the future after COVID-19, it is important to know that the trend of ever-expanding central bank balance sheets started during the last crisis — and that it was always likely to continue in the future.

The fact that central banks have been able to conjure funds from the ether in order to buy various assets from mortgage-backed securities (MBS) and Treasuries to corporate debt and equities is disconcerting. But it was highly effective, and I have long noted my expectations that it would likely occur again. After all, if it works, why stop now?

The Federal Reserve

In response to slow growth after the Great Recession, the U.S. Federal Reserve engaged in purchasing mortgage-backed securities as a means to push down mortgage rates and stimulate housing activity in the United States. The Fed also purchased Treasuries, which pushed down interest rates — even after the federal funds rate was set by the Federal Reserve at zero percent.

The Fed increased its balance sheet in 2008 from around $900 billion in January 2008 to around a peak of $4.5 trillion by January 2015. But the Fed did not buy equities or corporate bonds — although that is something they are now doing, effective March 2020, as a result of the COVID-19 pandemic.

Beginning in October 2017, the U.S. Fed began reducing its balance sheet in a formal policy of balance sheet reductions by reducing reinvestment of maturing mortgage-backed securities and Treasuries. However, unlike the European Central Bank's attempt to reduce its balance sheet between 2012 and 2014, the Fed deliberately planned a very slow pace of balance sheet reductions. It was due, in part, to the disastrous experience of the ECB that the Fed decided to be especially cautious in reducing the size of its own balance sheet.

But even the Fed's slow pace of balance sheet reduction engendered a U.S. business investment recession in 2019. So, the Fed reversed course in October 2019, re-expanding its balance sheet again, as you can see in Figure 7-1.

With the onset of COVID-19 risks, it accelerated the expansion.

The Future of Quantitative Easing

Expanding the Fed's balance sheet was highly effective at stimulating the U.S. economy, and for me that has always meant that the Fed would expand its balance sheet more in the future.

Janet Yellen even noted at the annual Kansas City Fed event in Jackson Hole, Wyoming, in 2016 that "I expect that forward guidance and asset purchases will remain important components of the Fed's policy toolkit." She further added that "Future policymakers may wish to explore the possibility of purchasing a broader range of assets."[1]

In recent weeks, as a response to COVID-19 pandemic risks for the entire economy, the Fed has expanded its asset purchases and essentially offered to back almost any investment grade debt.

Figure 7-1: Total Fed Balance Sheet Assets[2]

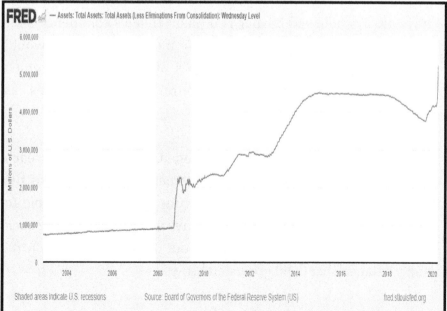

Plus, for now, there doesn't seem to be much downside. Globally, as long as all central banks are doing this, it may not drastically impact foreign exchange rates. After all, if everyone plays the game, it's tougher for there to be an outright winner — or loser. And they all want to play the quantitative easing game again if they can.

The Future Quantum State of the U.S. Economy

As we look ahead to the future of finance after COVID, we expect ever-greater expansions of central bank balance sheets. One of the things I often speak about is a risk that with each cyclical downturn in the future, central banks may continue to expand their balance sheets.

Indeed, with COVID-19 risks high, that is exactly what the Fed has announced.

I have always believed former Fed Chair Yellen's comments, so it has always seemed highly likely to me that the Fed would eventually need to diversify the kinds of assets it buys, which could include everything from corporate debt to equities, as other central banks have done.

Indeed, this is now what has happened. Of course, with each cycle, the central bank will become increasingly important as the buyer of last resort so that the U.S. economy becomes too big to fail. And as the U.S. Federal Reserve buys more assets during each downturn with money that it pulled out of nowhere, the central bank's balance sheet will grow and grow.

One potential worst-case scenario is where the central bank — after decades of cycles — eventually owns almost everything in the economy. And it will have paid for the debt, MBS, Treasuries, equities, and maybe even physical assets on its balance sheet with money it created — with money it didn't have in the first place.

This is effectively how we could have a quantum state of the economy, where the central bank owns everything with nothing. Then we would have a big problem.

I have often discussed and written about this risk, including in my book *The Future of Finance is Now* (2019).

The way in which central banks seek to instill confidence that they won't go down this path will be a critical priority in the decade ahead. And if they fail, this doomsday scenario could very well come to pass.

In the face of COVID-19, increased Fed balance sheet expansion and related actions have been critical for supporting the economy — and confidence in investment grade debt instruments. But the Fed may still buy more assets yet, further expanding its balance sheet to combat the economic risks of the COVID-19 pandemic. This means that — at least for the moment — the potential for a future quantum state of the economy appears not unlikely.

CHAPTER 8

THE FUTURE OF FISCAL POLICY

One of the biggest challenges for the future of finance is the rising U.S. national debt. Every economist, FOMC member, and Fed Chair warns about the negative impact high levels of debt are likely to have on long-term growth rates. But these warnings go largely unheeded, leaving dismal scientists to play Cassandra.

You could say that U.S. fiscal conservatism largely died with the 2017 tax cuts. And yet most politicians and economists supported the CARES Act, which is a $2.3 trillion bill designed to help the U.S. economy weather the storm of the COVID-19 pandemic.[1]

I, too, believed it necessary to push through a significant fiscal stimulus bill. After all, the U.S. economy in 2019 grew by $21.4 trillion (in current dollars) — or at about $1.8 trillion per month.[2]

That's a big number. And if the U.S. economy goes into a full shutdown for a month as a result of COVID-19, that's $1.8 trillion that would be lost forever. It can't really be recouped. It would just be lost. And the economic and human toll would be high.

Don't get me wrong. I believe that the unnecessary increase in deficit spending and the national debt in normal times — or during periods of solid growth — is a big risk. And one of the reasons it is such a risky action is that during times of economic crisis, fiscal policy is mustered to help combat the risks of a recession or depression.

But if we use all of our fiscal policy power during years of feast, what shall we do in years of famine?

Fortunately, interest rates are exceptionally low, and the Fed is using its balance sheet to keep those rates artificially low. This means that issuing more debt now is not as big a problem as it could be — or as big a problem as it will be in the future.

Nevertheless, let's face it: The U.S. national debt is a growing problem. At almost $23.2 trillion, the national debt is not a small sum.[3] And by the end of this year, the national debt could be $28 trillion or more.

That is a lot of debt!

As you can see in Figure 8-1, the pace at which the U.S. national debt is rising has accelerated. It took 205 years for the U.S. national debt to exceed $1 trillion, which happened in October 1981. But it then took less than five years for the national debt to double to $2 trillion in April 1986. The most recent doubling of the U.S. national debt occurred in the decade after the Great Recession. Hopefully the current slowdown will not cause it to double again.

Figure 8-1: Total U.S. Federal Debt[4]

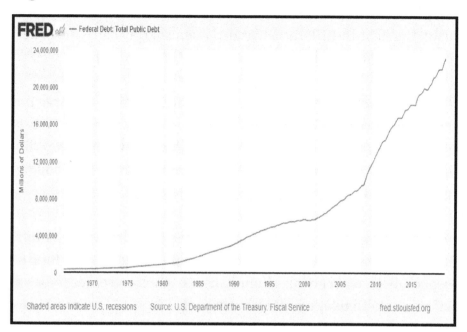

Figure 8-2: Total U.S. Federal Debt as a Percent of GDP[5]

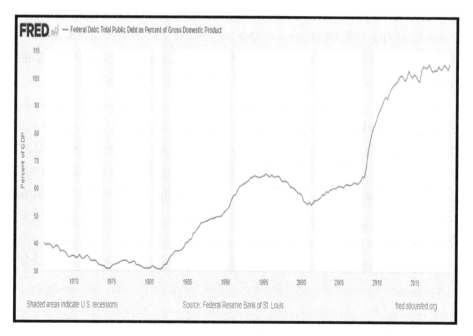

Although not as pronounced as the trend in total U.S. government debt, the debt-to-GDP ratio has also risen sharply since the onset of the Great Recession in December 2007 (Figure 8-2).

One major negative impact of a high national debt is the drag on potential future U.S. economic growth as measured by gross domestic product — or GDP. Plus, debt exposures can be exacerbated by compounding interest on already outstanding government debt.

For now, low interest rates all over the world have kept this specter at bay. But this could become a risk in the future, especially if central bank balance sheet expansion ceases to be as effective as stimulating economic growth.

Although some analysts are quick to note that the U.S. debt-to-GDP ratio is lower than other countries, it is also important to note that the U.S. economy is the largest in the world. This means that rising U.S. debt levels could make it more difficult for the global economy to absorb U.S. debt issuances over time.

Risks of Debt

As I noted in *The Dumpster Fire Election* last year, "the risk of recession would further increase the likelihood that the debt level and the debt-to-GDP ratio would rise between 2020 and 2024."

And entitlements are a major source of additional imminent debt.

Unfortunately, while the U.S. national debt is large, the unfunded financial obligations stemming from U.S. entitlements are much larger — and are likely to compound U.S. debt problems in coming years. Simply put, entitlements pose the greatest threat to future U.S. government debt levels — and U.S. economic growth.

Entitlements

U.S. entitlements, including Medicare, Medicaid, and Social Security, are financed by payroll taxes from workers. Payroll taxes are separate from income taxes, and while income tax rates have fallen on fiscal policy changes, payroll taxes are on a one-way trip higher. You see, entitlements are wildly underfunded.

All the sovereign debt in the world totals around $60 trillion.[6] That is the debt cumulatively held by all national governments in the world. But the size of unfunded U.S. entitlements might be more than three times that level. That's right: The unfunded, off-balance sheet obligations for Medicare, Medicaid, and Social Security could be $200 trillion.[7]

This level of off-balance sheet debt obligation existentially threatens the U.S. economy. The Heritage Foundation has taken calculations from the U.S. Congressional Budget Office about entitlements to create Figure 8-3, which looks quite catastrophic. Basically, by 2030, all U.S. tax revenue will be consumed by entitlements and the interest on the national debt. And these were the dismal calculations before the 2007 tax reform, additional budget deficits, and the 2020 CARES Act started increasing the national debt even more rapidly.

The Grandfather of U.S. Social Security

Part of the problem with entitlements stems from their origins. The U.S. Social Security Administration website credits Otto von Bismarck as the grandfather of U.S. entitlements.[8]

Bismarck's portrait is even on the U.S. Social Security Administration's website (Figure 8-4).

Bismarck was a powerful politician known for his use of *Realpolitik*, a political doctrine built on pragmatism to advance national self-interests. For him, entitlements were convenient and expedient. Unfortunately, that is no longer the case. Today, entitlements threaten to crush the U.S. economy with increased levels of debt. And without reform, they could decimate the U.S. workforce.

Figure 8-3: Tax Revenue Spent on Entitlements[9]

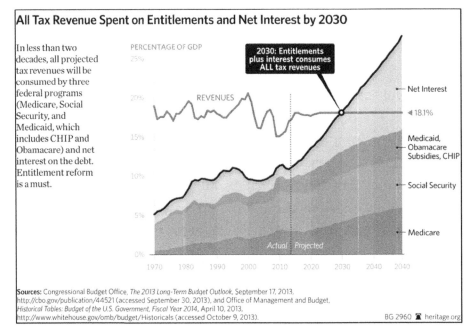

Bismarck's system was also sustainable. His system guaranteed a pension to German workers over 70, but the average life expectancy in Germany in the late 1880s was only 40.[10] In other words, so few people were expected to receive the benefits that the program's cost would be negligible.

Bismarck rigged entitlements to help crush his political opponents without having to pay out. But the current entitlement system in the United States is an unfunded off-balance sheet liability that threatens to crush the entire economy.

Plus, fixing entitlements presents a horrible dilemma as many Americans rely heavily on entitlements for income (Figure 8-5).

Figure 8-4: Grandfather of Social Security Otto von Bismarck[11]

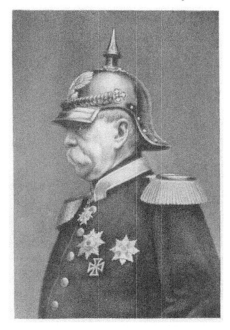

But how did this system break down? Bismarck had such a good thing going. What happened?

This can be answered in one word: demographics.

Demographics

U.S. population growth has slowed sharply, and this demographic shift appears unstoppable. Plus, as birthrates have fallen, life expectancy has also risen. This compounds the funding shortfalls for entitlements. Worse still: No president, senator, or congressman can change U.S. demographics. This is bigger than one person.

Figure 8-5: Expected Importance of Social Security[12]

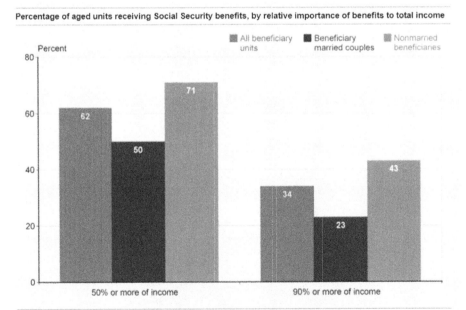

SOURCE: SSA calculations from the March 2016 Annual Social and Economic Supplement to the Current Population Survey.
NOTE: An aged unit is a married couple living together or a nonmarried person, which also includes persons who are separated or married but not living together.

And its discussion is unlikely to be anywhere near the 2020 presidential election — and other coming elections as well.

Population growth in the United States has fallen from annual rates of over 1.5 percent per year during the 1950s and early 1960s to just 0.7 percent since 2011.[13]

Some of this slowing in population growth is due to a decline in the U.S. fertility rate. In general, fertility rates have been dropping globally, but according to demographer Jonathan Last, the U.S. fertility rate is still relatively high at 1.93.[14]

However, even though the U.S. total fertility rate is relatively high compared to other industrialized nations, it is below the 2.1 percent "golden number" required to maintain a population, according to Last.[15]

This is a huge problem for maintaining entitlements. After all, the entitlement system worked really well in 1940, when there were 159.4 workers per beneficiary (Figure 8-6). But it is more challenging since that number fell to only 2.8 in 2013.

Plus, it is likely to fall to 2 workers per beneficiary by 2040.[16]

Entitlements are under siege from both sides: The birthrate has fallen — and life expectancy has risen.

In addition to lower birthrates, U.S. life expectancy has doubled since Bismarck implemented entitlements in Germany in 1889 — from around 40 years to above 80 years. Plus, the age at which people receive U.S. entitlements benefits has actually been lowered from 70 to 65. On top of a significantly larger population being eligible to receive entitlements, the medical costs required to support an aging population have also risen.

Everything might be OK — if U.S. population growth were extremely robust. But it is not.

Figure 8-6: Ratio of Workers to Social Security Beneficiaries[17]

Year	Covered Workers (in thousands)	Beneficiaries (in thousands)	Ratio
1940	35,390	222	159.4
1945	46,390	1,106	41.9
1950	48,280	2,930	16.5
1955	65,200	7,563	8.6
1960	72,530	14,262	5.1
1965	80,680	20,157	4.0
1970	93,090	25,186	3.7
1975	100,200	31,123	3.2
1980	113,656	35,118	3.2
1985	120,565	36,650	3.3
1990	133,672	39,470	3.4
1995	141,446	43,107	3.3
2000	155,295	45,166	3.4
2005	159,081	48,133	3.3
2010	156,725	53,398	2.9
2013	163,221	57,471	2.8

Plus, the current administration is pushing hard to reduce illegal immigration to the United States. While this can have some benefits for society and the economy in some ways, it can also reduce population growth and lower the average U.S. birthrate.

Population growth has slowed to less than half the rate seen during the baby boom years, and the total U.S. fertility rate is below the "golden number" that is required to maintain a population. As Last notes, "Social Security is, in essence, a Ponzi scheme. Like all Ponzi schemes, it works just fine — so long as the intake of new participants continues to increase."[18] Unfortunately, entitlements are nearing a breaking point.

A big problem with slowing birthrates is the manifestation of a shrinking tax base at the same time that unfunded financial obligations are rising. This means that the unfunded $200 trillion or more in future entitlements payments will be borne by an increasingly smaller proportion of workers in the population.

In the longer term, declines in birthrates, increased longevity, rising healthcare costs, falling labor force participation rates, and overincentivized automation are likely to accelerate and exacerbate the problems of the U.S. national defined benefits programs known as entitlements — programs that worked best financially when the age at which one received benefits exceeded life expectancy by 30 years.

But the entitlements system was ignored during the 2016 presidential election, during the 2017 tax reform, and in the 2018 midterms. And it is being ignored now in the 2020 election cycle.

COVID-19 Implications for Fiscal Policy

As in other areas, the COVID-19 pandemic has exposed systemic weaknesses already present. The national debt and entitlements risks were already in play before the federal government had to pull the trigger on a $2.3 trillion fiscal policy bailout to keep the economy alive during what has become essentially a mandated shutdown.

The future of fiscal policy looks like one of additional fiscal stimulus, ever-higher debt levels, and unaddressed entitlements. On top of those risks, there is also a chance that the free money individuals are sent during this crisis could become a permanent political fixture.

And it could even become part of the broader discourse on universal basic income — or UBI.

Universal basic income (UBI) is the notion that everyone will be paid a flat salary, regardless of whether or not they work. And the biggest problem with universal basic income is that we simply cannot afford it. U.S. entitlement obligations, which could be as high as $200 trillion, make a further, permanent expansion of ongoing U.S. budgetary obligations for UBI virtually impossible.

But because of the policies enacted in response to COVID-19, UBI could become a permanent fixture. That remains to be seen. But a future of more debt and unaddressed entitlements seems far more certain. And even without UBI, those are sufficient grounds to be concerned about long-term growth rates for the U.S. economy.

Hopes for Future Fiscal Prudence

Massive unfunded off-balance sheet debt obligations — à la entitlements — could eventually subvert stable Western financial systems, eradicating economic growth and introducing destabilizing factors that could subvert democracy itself.

Some reading this may see my views here as hyperbole. And believe me, I wish they were. But sadly, they are not. And on a global scale, these problems are even worse.

The problems we have been ignoring could drastically impact economic and business growth expectations globally — especially in consumer-driven service economies, where drastically reduced incomes of retirees could dovetail with significantly increased payroll taxes for prime-age workers. For the future of the economy and financial markets, the impact of these risks cannot be understated.

I understand that in the face of risks associated with total economic shutdown and systemic public health collapse, this is not a time to implement fiscal austerity. It is, however, a time to reflect on how we might plan to be more fiscally responsible and prudent once this pandemic is behind us — so that we can act even more quickly the next time a crisis like this arises.

Of course, we may not see future fiscal prudence either.

But one can hope.

CHAPTER 9

THE FUTURE OF REAL ESTATE

The real estate industry could be significantly impacted by the aftershocks of COVID-19. There are six different ways that I see a high potential for this to play out:
— **Reduced commercial office demand.**
— **Reduced retail space demand.**
— **Risk of housing oversupply and price declines.**
— **High risks to real estate in tourism-centric areas.**
— **Likely tradeoff preference for space vs. proximity.**
— **More demand for warehouse and distribution centers.**

First, there's a potential that people may increasingly telecommute and work remotely. I've discussed this in other chapters here in the book, so I won't dive back into that in too much detail. But the main point is, if more people are working remotely, companies won't need as much office space, and those companies will save money by not paying for office space.

Of course, if you happen to be the one who owns the office buildings, this is likely to be a source of financial pain.

It seems likely to me that some high-end commercial real estate could be converted into hotels, condos, or mixed-use real estate. This stems from a likely key influencing factor: If people continue to work remotely at levels anywhere near those seen during the COVID-19 pandemic, we will likely find that we have far too much commercial real estate for offices — especially expensive real estate in areas with high urban density.

The second big impact that we could see as an aftershock of COVID-19 would be in the retail real estate space. We have been seeing a transition to e-commerce for some time. But that has become more pronounced — and more economically critical — during the COVID-19 pandemic.

As a result, we may find that a lot of small mom-and-pop businesses, family restaurants, small service businesses, and small retail shops completely shut down and go out of business as in the economic aftermath of the COVID-19 pandemic.

The pandemic has had a particularly notorious impact on service businesses because these are high-touch businesses, and yet that is completely anathema to the notion of flattening the curve and trying to do your part to reduce transmission. High-touch businesses like massage therapy, nail salons, and hair salons require very close personal touch, and that's not something that is consistent with flattening the curve and reducing transmission of COVID-19 during a pandemic. Furthermore, since some of these businesses are quite small, they may struggle to survive — even if they can access some of the funds in the $2.3 trillion CARES Act.

As such I expect a lot of small restaurants and small businesses will shut down, never to reopen. Additionally, the reliance on e-commerce is likely to be much stronger after the events of COVID-19, and given the increased reliance on e-commerce I expect that retail real estate is likely to lose even greater value moving forward, with entire chains likely to fail during the post-pandemic period.

Another big change — the third big change — I expect is the potential for real estate residential markets to take a hit. If jobs do not come back and businesses fail, there will be evictions, there will be bankruptcies, there will be mortgage failures, and even though the government can help to bridge some of the lending and some of the gaps to prevent widespread national mortgage failures, there are going to be some areas where people owning houses will default on their mortgages.

People who will be upside down pretty quickly on their mortgages might try to sell them quickly. Therefore, it seems likely that we may see a lot of houses come on the market for sale at once. Since home prices are a function of supply and demand, you might find there's a massive supply of people trying to get out of their homes, which could depress prices of homes that people are trying very hard to sell quickly. This is also something that could impact the financial health of the economy. I discussed this risk at length in the "The Future of Finance" chapter in this book.

As a fourth expectation, I am very concerned about areas with high levels of tourism like Las Vegas, Orlando, and New Orleans.

Casinos and theme parks have been forcibly shut down, because high tourist areas present high risks of COVID-19 exposure. If there is a prolonged COVID-19 breakout, these cities will likely suffer disproportionately. Furthermore, even if the COVID-19 pandemic were to end quickly, tourism dollars would likely be very tight. Disposable incomes might be slow to recover and if that's the case, we could likely see these major tourist hubs continue to suffer, even after people are legally allowed to return to them.

The fifth important dynamic we expect is an increase in the preference for more residential real estate *space* over a closer *proximity to work*. By this, I mean that we may see home buyers begin to demonstrate a more pronounced preference for larger, suburban homes over condos close to urban centers.

Many people were predicting greater trends in U.S. urbanization for most of the past 15 years or so. But this pandemic may have a couple of significant impacts that reverse that trend. First, the remote work experience may change people's perceptions about the value of space. If people are working remotely with their entire families in close quarters — rather than going to an office regularly — population-level preferences are likely to shift toward more space.

Furthermore, the risks of hoarding, food shortages, and public health contagion risks are likely to be heightened in more densely populated urban areas. This, too, seems likely to impact people's preferences for the suburbs or more rural areas over cities — and major urban centers.

This seems especially likely for families that have adults working remotely as their kids are going to school online. If everybody's going to school and work under the same roof, people are certainly going to show preferences for more space, rather than to be in a condo right near the office they never go to or the school their kids never go to.

There's a sixth and final dynamic for the future of real estate as a result of COVID-19: a likely increase in demand for warehouse and distribution center square footage. The critical nature of the supply chain and the importance of e-commerce are likely to drive this demand.

For real estate, these six big changes seem likely in the years ahead — and beyond. Some of these dynamics may not be new, but COVID-19 has revealed and accelerated some of these changes in perception and value.

CHAPTER 10

THE FUTURE OF AGRICULTURE

Agriculture could be significantly impacted by the economic and socioeconomic dynamics of COVID-19. After all, widespread food shortages, especially shortages in fresh foods, like fruits, vegetables, eggs, meats, and cheeses, are likely to inspire more people to go into the agriculture profession.

The big takeaway here is that for almost all Americans alive today, food has been generally taken for granted. But now we've seen a reawakening — a reemergence — of concerns around foodstuffs. That will have a real impact in what people might look at as important investable ideas. And it could impact what careers people choose as a result of this pandemic.

There may also be increased investor interest in indoor food production warehouses, indoor grow centers, and distributed agricultural facilities for plants as well as lab-grown meats. I expect we are likely to see increased funding for labs to grow meat as well as multistoried hydroponic facilities to generate food like vegetables and fish.

A Food Wakeup Call

Food is at the bottom of Maslow's hierarchy of needs. It's something that most Americans have taken for granted for some time. It's something most people assumed there would be no issues with — especially because the United States is a major exporter of food. Fortunately, the United States produces more food than it consumes. But supply chains have been negatively impacted, and the inability to get fresh food and certain foodstuffs has had a real impact.

Those disruptions could inspire people to do more at-home farming. In fact, I personally know people who are putting in gardens at their houses as a result of the COVID-19 pandemic. I know others who are getting set up with chickens or other livestock in order to have some of the fresh food they want at the house.

And this isn't a fringe phenomenon. In recent weeks, I have had numerous phone calls with CEOs and executives of both public and private companies, on which we have shared tips and tricks about where to order food online that could not be found at local markets, including cheeses, meats, fruits, vegetables, and fish.

Although there are always people in almost every country in the world who struggle with access to basic necessities, including food. But these are things that I never thought would be an issue for the population at large in the 21st century. It had not previously occurred to me that if I wanted eggs, I better get some chickens. It is scary to think that this may be the new paradigm for how some business professionals need to think about food.

Perhaps the most surprising thing about these dynamics is that this is no longer just a consideration for people trying to live off the grid. This is now something to consider for anyone who wants to be sure of their food supply.

Going forward, it seems very likely that we would see more interest in the agricultural space for investing, careers, and national security than we have seen in a long time.

I also think a major change for agriculture is going to include much more widespread use of food delivery from supermarkets. For most of the past century, it was really only some elderly people who had their food delivered. I remember my Great Aunt Bertha had food delivered to her in the 1980s. And I know it was common for older people long before that.

And man, did those older folks have the right idea!

In recent years, there have been a slew of apps developed to help people get groceries they need delivered. Based on the use of such apps during the COVID-19 pandemic, I think you're going to see more widespread adoption of their use permanently, as a direct result of people having been forced to use these various food delivery apps.

As for jobs, there has been a massive decline in the part of the U.S. labor force dedicated to agriculture. In fact, agricultural jobs were close to a majority of the labor force in the mid-1800s. But now, the percent of the workforce in agriculture is close to less than 1 percent in the United States.

Looking forward, I expect that we are going to see more people go into farming in the next few years — and potentially throughout this decade.

That fear of not being able to get food and the panic of going to a market that doesn't have food is going to weigh on people going forward. This is likely to be especially true for younger people who are planning out their careers.

Maybe they're in middle school or high school or college, and they're trying to think about what they want to do with their lives. And having these experiences during the COVID-19 pandemic of being unable to find the food they want is going to impact some of their major life decisions.

Because I was born in the 1970s, I recall images and stories of life in the former Soviet Union, where people were unable to get toilet paper and food. The fact that this was America in 2020 is shocking to me. And these kinds of things are going to cast a long shadow over people's careers and lives in a material way.

As people debate what are essential workers and what are nonessential workers, one thing is not up for debate: agriculture. Because it is the epitome of an essential industry. Without food, we have nothing.

CHAPTER 11

THE FUTURE OF SUPPLY CHAIN

Paper product and fresh food shortages in the United States resulting from the COVID-19 pandemic came as a surprise to many people. But as a result of this dynamic, many people have also come to recognize the importance of the U.S. supply chain, the global supply chain, supply chain and material handling industries, and the challenges of the last mile.

The COVID-19 pandemic experience was jostling for many Americans, and there are significant changes to supply chain that I expect we will likely see in the post-pandemic period.

First, the vulnerability of U.S. and global supply chains have been revealed. I believe that it should now be clear to many that disruptions in the supply chain can occur anywhere in the global economy and that the negative impacts of supply chain disruptions can be exacerbated when inventories are thin. In truth, it should now be clear that the long-term trends of simultaneously spreading out supply chains while maintaining low inventories can be a recipe for disaster.

Second, medical supplies and medical devices that had long been taken for granted as easily accessible have been revealed to be sometimes difficult to obtain. Hearing from medical professionals looking to reuse previously single-use personal protection equipment (PPE) or medical devices is scary. In the future, the medical supply chain is likely to be recognized as more critical. And policies are likely to be enacted to reduce medical supply chain risks.

Third, the supply chain of the U.S. economy is something that almost everyone now more clearly understands. The words "supply chain" were barely uttered in business schools in the 1990s and early 2000s. But now, supply chain needs to be a top-of-mind topic for every executive, every politician, every leader, and every consumer.

Where our goods come from, how they get to us, and when they get to us are critical issues that people can no longer ignore. And it may be somewhat of a near-term challenge to instill great confidence in a supply chain that is spread very thin — and spread globally.

The Bullwhip Effect
When the supply chain suffers a shock of demand, this pulls supply forward; thin inventories and supplies throughout the entire supply chain can be pulled forward to the source of end consumption rapidly. The impact on the supply side is a rush to produce more. But it still takes time for those goods to move through the supply chain.

But as more supplies are dispatched to meet the surge in demand, you are likely to end up with a lumpy supply chain, with significantly more supply bunched up at points in the supply chain — or you may fund a glut of supply ends up at the final point of consumption at a future point in time.

Simply put, sometimes the supply chain just can't go any faster. And when it speeds up, you may end up with bunched-up excess supply at points in the chain or at the traditional point of final consumption. This result is what supply chain practitioners call a bullwhip effect. And it's called a bullwhip effect because a bullwhip is a long whip that with just a tiny flick of your wrist can create a big and loud crack at the end of it.

Of course, the risk of a bullwhip effect isn't a sufficient reason to abandon the attempt to push supply chains forward in times of crisis — especially when it comes to critical items that have been disrupted, like fresh foods, paper products, toilet paper, medical equipment, and personal protection equipment (PPE), including gloves and masks.

Part of the problem wasn't just a surge in demand. Some of it was tight supply. In other words, inventories were low.

The reason?

Many firms have been able to increase their profitability by lowering their inventories over time, but this strategy has now been revealed to be a sometimes risky one.

Changes in Medical and PPE Supply Chains

It is very difficult to have both a thin supply chain and very large distances across your supply chain. In fact, very thin inventories plus a very long supply chain can be a recipe for disaster during times of disaster, which is exactly what we have seen as a result of the COVID-19 pandemic.

As a result of this experience, we are likely to see a future shift of policies and strategies to favor more robust inventories spread across supply chains. This could include some regulatory incentives and/or mandates related to the manufacture, storage, and inventory of medical and PPE supplies in the future.

It is also quite conceivable that there could be a regulatory or policy attempt to completely reshape the entire supply chains for medical equipment and PPE, so that more goods are produced within the United States or the USMCA/NAFTA region. Shortening the distances of supply chains can help counteract the risk that accompanies supply chain inventories that have been spread thin. And global supply chain risks are inherently greater than domestic supply chain risks because of the distance, number of parties, and regulations involved.

Risks to Restaurants

People may also reevaluate the stability of food supply chains in the future. This presents some risks to the hospitality industry, restaurant businesses, tourism, and other industries. Food has traditionally been distributed through two main channels: a commercial channel that feeds into restaurants and other places to eat, as well as a consumer channel to supermarkets.

As a result of the changes and regulations, including "shelter in place" mandates and quarantines, people are now consuming more of their food from supermarkets at home.

The longer the COVID-19 pandemic lasts, the more difficult it will be for restaurants and other non-markets that sell food. After all, if this disruption persists for a protracted period of time, the food supply chain is likely to become adaptive, such that fresh foods no longer feed into commercial channels. In short, these commercial foods could be redirected to supermarkets, which would actually create even greater problems for restoring business to restaurants and other places to eat.

This presents a near-term risk of change in food supply chains. And while this change may help solve some supermarket food supply chain issues and shortages of fresh food products, like eggs, milk, cheese, meats, vegetables, fruits, and other perishables, it could create corporate problems for restaurants that wish to reopen. After all, if supply chains shift on a more sustained basis, and the source of end demand changes, this could make it almost impossible for restaurants to open again. After all, they might then have trouble securing fresh food, toilet paper, dishwashing solution, cleaning supplies, and other paper products.

The Importance of Supply Chain for Stability
Stability of the economy depends very much on goods and services getting to where they are needed. And a disruption of those goods presents not just risks to the economy but actual risks to people and potentially to national security.

Fortunately, in the United States, we are net exporters of food. But other countries are not so lucky. And food disruptions in other countries could become more dire.

When talking about people and how they live, Berthold Brecht, the playwright of *The Threepenny Opera*, wrote the line "Erst kommt das Fressen, dann kommt die Moral." It translates roughly to "First comes the feeding, then come the morals."

In other words, if people do not have access to food, this could destabilize an entire economy.

As the COVID-19 situation was evolving, I was doing some Department of Defense work, and multiple discussions I had revolved around the hope that the supply chain for food and other basic goods was as secure as people had claimed. So far, that seems to have been the case, which is quite fortunate.

However, if our supply chain were not to have been so secure either for food or basic goods, we could have seen the entire stability of the country fall apart. This could have presented a significant stabilization risk at the national level — and it may yet still. But so far, it has not.

Not far behind food are medical devices, medical equipment, and PPE. As I mentioned above, I expect that we may likely see shifting regulatory or financial incentives applied to medical supply chains in the future. These, too, are essential items. And the critical impact of a shortage in these goods is unlikely to go unnoticed by national security professionals.

Awareness of Supply Chains

One final big impact of the recent COVID-19 pandemic is that people are likely to be more aware of supply chains. And they may be less likely to run down their own "at-home" inventories of food, paper products, cleaning products, and other goods.

In other words, people might keep more things at their house.

There's an old nursery rhyme about Mother Hubbard and her cupboard. As you may recall, her cupboard was bare.

Because people have been able to get goods with relative ease for some time, people did not worry about what was in their cupboard. After all, you don't mind if you have a bare cupboard if you can get whatever food you need to your house in under 20 minutes.

But in the COVID-19 pandemic situation, people found supply chains disrupted while their cupboards were also bare. This problem became exacerbated by the risk that people might need to stay in their homes for extended periods. People had to restock their cupboards rapidly because they had low in-home inventories and they expected a rise in demand as alternative sources of food (e.g., restaurants) became less viable. This is what contributed to the bullwhip effect for food and paper products.

The food supply chain as well as the supply chain for paper products demand was shifted from being consumed at home *and away* to solely being consumed at home. And there were no reserve foodstuffs; there was no back of house.

Mother Hubbard's cupboard was bare everywhere, and people had to react quickly.

At the same time, the consumption of paper products and food shifted from a mix of commercial and residential consumption to almost exclusively residential consumption. In the future, we will want more secure supply chains. But it remains to be seen if people will prevent their cupboards from going bare again after the COVID-19 pandemic passes.

Expectations Summary
The expectations I've shared in this chapter seem to be reasonable futurist expectations. After all, we have now revealed a few problems because of the COVID-19 pandemic. But we do know that the fundamental drivers of change are likely to be impacted by basic fundamentals:
— People always want to have access to food.
— People want to always feel secure in their access to medical care.
— Society only functions if people have access to that food and that medical care and they feel secure in it.

This is why I believe we could see additional financial incentives or regulatory incentives from the government that shore up the supply chain in the future.

CHAPTER 12

THE FUTURE OF MEDIA

COVID-19 has magnified weaknesses and problems across industries. This is also true for media and social media. How people have responded to COVID-19 news and online posts does not bode well.

And it's primarily because of false consensus bias.

For some time, social media has been fostering false consensus bias, which is the perception that what you believe is what everyone believes.

Essentially, this happens when you believe that your view is that of the consensus — even if you have fringe beliefs. This happens because even if only a handful of people on your Facebook feed agree with you, social media feeds optimize for interactions, which leads to individually optimized information feeds and personalized information curation. This, in turn, fosters a feeling that everyone believes what you do. Or, more specifically, what you and your peers believe to be true — is truth.

The whole experience of COVID-19 has been quite the bugaboo for the media. This is a situation that wasn't fully understood at first. And to a certain degree, it is still not fully understood.

There has been a steady stream of changing and evolving data about the situation. And this evolving situation dynamic did not occur in a bubble. It occurred against the backdrop of increased subjectivist realities.

Highly individualized perceptions of importance and truth related to facts that stem from curation and feed into consensus bias are the backdrop. It's part of the reason some people say that we are in a post-truth era.

This stems from the hyper-individualized nature of social media, which has fostered sub-national identities and subjectivist truths, among other things. So, even though COVID-19 became a full-blown pandemic, the evolving situation in which it became exponential had actually started very small.

The story was managed differently by various media sources, and it was perceived differently by viewers and across social media. Skepticism about how believable certain media or social media are contributed to some confusion.

There were so many unknowns, but people still rushed to become experts in COVID-19 quickly. After all, the importance of pandemic risk is so great that forecasters, futurists, analysts, strategists, executives, and politicians had to have a perspective on the topic.

Based on some of the recent political interference and psychological operations foreign actors have implemented using Facebook and other social media, this outcome is not unexpected.

After all, confusion stemming from a lack of real information led to the rise of false expertise and festering skepticism buttressed by adherence to subjectivist truth.

The media has always lived by the phrase "if it bleeds, it leads." This is the idea that the more gruesome or shocking or horrifying a story is, the more important it is — and the higher the billing would be in print or television media. And when it comes to bleeding and leading, almost nothing bleeds quite like a disease that starts in a wildlife market in China. This is especially true for a Western audience for which the images of the market include never-before-seen exotic animals that may have somehow engendered the COVID-19 pandemic.

Some people took the COVID-19 pandemic risks hyper-seriously well before the data showed that perhaps it should be. And yet, even as I write this, there are many people who do not view this as a serious situation.

This is the cost of consensus bias.

And this is not the last critical time that it will rear its ugly head. I expect subjectivist truth, subjectivist realities, subnational identity, and hyper-individualized information feeds will lead to further problems of unwarranted skepticism in the future. And each time this happens, there could be deleterious consequences.

Looking at the future of media after COVID-19 does not make me terribly optimistic. The more national identity is fractured, the greater the risk is that it could be exploited by bad actors. Since there will not be any shortage of bad actors anytime soon, this presents significant risks to societal cohesion over time.

As in other areas, COVID-19 has already revealed things that were hidden in plain sight. In terms of media and social media, the things that were lying beneath the surface — the potential for consensus bias, risk of psy-ops, and subjectivist truth — were not positive ones.

CHAPTER 13

THE FUTURE OF INTERNATIONAL RELATIONS

International relations will be significantly impacted by COVID-19. The relationship between the United States and China was already strained by a trade war that started in early 2018 and continued throughout 2018 and 2019. Some of the key U.S. tariffs still remain in place.

Now, with the COVID-19 pandemic, there are added tensions stemming from how the novel coronavirus spread.

President Trump's insistence on still calling COVID-19 "the Chinese virus" indicates that there is a high level of tension just below the surface. And it does not seem as if the struggle between China and the United States for global economic, political, and military hegemony will in any way be softened by recent developments.

In fact, it appears as if COVID-19 may sow more seeds of discontent along with increased tension between the two competing nations.

The fact that COVID-19 is a worldwide pandemic is a tricky thing from an international relations perspective. On the one hand, there is a tragically massive downside, including the human toll in terms of illness, suffering, death, and the risk of recession.

But if COVID-19 were only in one country, that could be quite a bit more challenging for that country's geopolitical standing. For example, if the United States were the only country that had COVID-19 while all other countries did not, it would be more difficult to manage from an American perspective. Such a risk could in turn present stabilization problems, and it could adversely affect the United States' ability to maintain and project its position in the world. In other words, there is a real risk that COVID-19 could engender an asymmetric negative geopolitical impact on a country that is solely afflicted if other countries are not.

The awareness of this kind of risk is perhaps one of the reasons that there could be lingering resentment between the United States and China. After all, some argue, this virus was able to spread globally after starting in Wuhan province.

These kinds of statements and sentiments present risks that even after the COVID-19 pandemic passes, there could be changes in how countries manage information. And it could impact how much trust there is between countries related to critical issues like pandemics. In short, there are risks that trust could be eroded. And one of the most important cornerstones of international relations is trust.

Without trust, you cannot have a positive development in relations between two international actors. And trust seems to be in short supply given recent COVID-19 developments.

On a global scale, risks to medical supply chains have also been exposed as a real risk for the safety of the American people, and given past preferences by the president for tariffs, it seems likely that more tariffs may ensue. Now, in the same way that the U.S. Section 232 tariffs on steel and aluminum were introduced to shore up supply chains of domestic metals production for materiel, it seems likely that there may be additional medical device tariffs to prevent the supply chain problems and economic chaos that the COVID-19 pandemic outbreak created.

It is important to remember that tariffs are something the president can implement unilaterally. This is a topic I explored in depth in my book *Midterm Economics* (2018). As such, if President Trump is reelected — or perhaps even before the 2020 presidential elections — he may seek to use tariffs to change and influence the future U.S. supply chain of medical devices and PPE as critical materials that need to be manufactured in the United States. Moreover, this tension between the United States and China is likely to lead to a bifurcated set of global supply chains further pulling more manufacturing out of China.

This could elevate the tensions. And although it is unlikely to put the United States and China on a "destined for war" footing, it is still likely to be a contributing factor for potential further erosion in relations between the countries that could lead to increasingly risky outcomes.[1]

Beyond the most immediate trade and manufacturing job concerns, it is also possible that manufacturing companies that are at risk of being isolated for protracted periods from the United States' end market may also independently begin to reshape their supply chains to manufacture more goods in the United States or the USMCA region.

This means that once the COVID-19 pandemic has passed, there may be more materials and goods manufacturing in the United States. And tensions between the United States and China could rise even further as the economic superpower proxy war continues.

CHAPTER 14

THE FUTURE OF NATIONAL SECURITY

The COVID-19 pandemic has opened the aperture in many ways, revealing open secrets and overlooked risks — for our society, our economy, and our security.

For national security, the COVID-19 pandemic has exposed the importance of being vigilant with our borders. And it highlights the risks of overly thin supply chains, as well as the potential downside of being dependent on the global supply chain for critical goods, like medical supplies, medical devices, basic necessities, and PPE, including gloves and masks.

Supply Chain as National Security Risk

Overly thin levels of inventory as well as long supply chains present risks to national security in the United States. As I mentioned in Chapter 11, most corporate entities have run their supply chain inventories exceptionally low. This thin level of supply produces risks, as does the geographic distance between trade partners, which introduces a lag time between which goods can be ordered and received.

As we have seen, this has been critical for medical devices and PPE. Trade risks were already a national security issue related to metals for materiel in the United States, which was the critical driving factor behind the implementation of the U.S. Section 232 tariffs on aluminum and steel. Additionally, the Section 301 tariffs highlighted risks to U.S. national security from Chinese threats to U.S. intellectual property.

And now, because of COVID-19, PPE and medical devices are on the hot list too. As a result, the U.S.-China trade war is likely to heat up from current levels, because risks that were previously considered somewhat fringe are now likely to be accepted as national security risks on a bipartisan basis.

In other words, both Democrats and Republicans may now come to see having critical goods, including metals for materiel, PPE for healthcare, foodstuffs, and paper products as important for maintaining civil order. In some respects, maintaining a secure supply chain is inherently difficult when the goods come from a country that is too far away for the goods to arrive quickly.

That realization is now going to receive more airtime — more talking space and room for discourse. So, we may very well see in the near term that both Democrats and Republicans will trip over themselves in order to support the idea of securing supply chains for critical medical devices, PPE equipment, foodstuffs, paper products, and pharmaceuticals to prevent the loss of American lives in the future — and to minimize the potential disruption or devastation of the American economy in the event of another pandemic.

After all, one of the big reasons we need to slow the spread of COVID-19 in the United States and "flatten the curve" is because there are not enough doctors, nurses, hospitals, ventilators, gloves, masks, or other equipment. If we could at least get the equipment piece under control, that may be something that could protect the economy and the American people in the future.

Risk of Exploitation
The COVID-19 outbreak has also revealed that the United States can be exploited in a pandemic-type event. Furthermore, if the United States could have been solely targeted it would have threatened national security significantly. Alternatively, if the United States could have been deceived into believing that flattening the curve could be beneficial — even when it was not — that, too, could have presented a risk.

This experience also reveals the vulnerability of the American public to media and social media messaging and potential manipulation around topics that may or may not be valid. This is part of my discussion about the risk of psychological operations (psy-ops) and subjectivist truth in Chapter 12.

In short, the United States from a national security perspective may very well wish to more firmly shore up technology, healthcare, medical, food, consumables, and other supply chains in order to ensure maximum stability for the United States over time. Additionally, COVID-19 has inadvertently revealed that a pandemic-level bio attack on the United States could be beyond economically devastating.

If adversaries of the United States were to implement such an attack, they could pair such action with social media and traditional media psy-ops for maximum disruption, political destabilization, and economic devastation in a way that could completely destabilize the United States as an entity for at least a brief period of time.

These kinds of risks may sound extreme. But we have also seen foodstuffs run low. And we have seen the American populace have to quarantine themselves at home.

On the policy side, the Fed is massively expanding its balance sheet by potentially adding $4 trillion. And fiscal policy stimulus in the CARES Act involved a $2.3 trillion package.

These policy actions alone underscore how expensive not being prepared really is.

If we were to, for a moment, consider the cost to have just produced more ventilators, masks, and gloves — and if we had simply educated more doctors and nurses, those costs would have likely been infinitesimal compared to the potentially $6 trillion-plus in policy support taken in order to prevent a collapse of the entire U.S. economy.

Those are things that people who work in the diplomatic core, international relations, and national security would very likely prefer not to consider.

Noise Framework

When I considered the importance of the COVID-19 pandemic for national security, I created what I call the NOISE framework, which examines some of the most important factors that contribute to national security and political stability.

Here is the NOISE framework, and the five critical factors that contribute to national security and political stability:

Necessities — *Food, Water, Power, Shelter, Safety*

Occupations — *Jobs, Vocations, and Hobbies*

Information — *Access to Accurate, Complete Information*

Systems — *Financial, Healthcare, Transportation, Education*

External — *International Relations, Military, Supply Chain, Trade*

As you can see, **first come the necessities**, which I have included as food, water, shelter, and safety. If people do not have these, then there are easily risks of political instability.

If these factors are stable, then a country or economy is likely to remain on an even keep. In the most recent experience of the COVID-19 pandemic, concerns about safety and food emerged. Maintaining the U.S. supply chain and basic services as well as utilities (like power and water) is critical.

Second are occupations. These stem from the notion that people — at the population level — need things to do. Can people be retired and do essentially nothing? Yes, of course. But as a nation, people need jobs, vocations, and hobbies. They just need to be doing something.

The need for this stabilizing force is tied to the notion that idle hands are the devil's workshop. This became a critical issue during the COVID-19 pandemic outbreak, as people were forced to "shelter in place." Some people could still work, but others were concerned about their jobs. This is why the CARES Act was so important. Because even if people cannot work, they need to know their chance of still having jobs will remain high after the pandemic ends.

The third element of stability is information. Information is not opinion. And real information is critical for maintaining order and keeping people calm — and aligned with the same interests. Under information, I have included sharing accurate and complete information. The risks here are misinformation, disinformation, psy-ops, opinion presented as fact, and subjectivist truth, when the truth is, in fact, objective.

Fourth are systems. National security depends on the proper functioning of a number of critical systems, including the financial system, the healthcare system, the transportation system, and the education system. All of these have been disrupted or are at risk of being disrupted by the COVID-19 pandemic.

The fifth element of national security stability is the external. This includes international relations, the existence and ability to deploy the military, the global supply chain, and trade. Fortunately, some of these core elements, like international relations and the military, have not yet been disrupted by the COVID-19 pandemic. But the global supply chain and trade have.

When considering the NOISE framework, it's easy to see how the COVID-19 pandemic has actually threatened all of these different pillars of national security and political stability in one way or another. And these risks justify the Fed's drastic action to support the credit markets, the federal government passage of the $2.3 trillion CARES Act to preserve jobs, the daily briefings about COVID-19 directly from White House staff and Trump administration leaders to share information, and why some supply chain regulations and laws may change in the future — especially with regard to medical devices, medical equipment, medications, and PPE equipment.

The COVID-19 pandemic threatened to push U.S. national security to the brink. But we have held the line so far because of significant and swift action from a wide swatch of vested parties.

But this won't be the last time this kind of risk appears. So, shoring up risks in advance could prove critical —especially because the next time might not be an accident. The next time, we could be a target. I suspect that the future of national security for years to come will focus on improving strategic preparedness for tail end events like the COVID-19 pandemic.

Manufacturing Companies and National Security

In addition to broad-based national security risks that have been revealed by the COVID-19 pandemic, there are also risks associated with disruption to national security vendors.

Some companies that produce goods for national security uses, like airplane manufacturers and airplane parts manufacturers, could find themselves suffering from challenging economic and business conditions as part of the slowdown in air travel.

While this is a second-order impact of the COVID-19 pandemic, it is a critical issue of primary importance for national security entities. Looking ahead, national security organizations will need to more aggressively monitor economic and business risks of critical vendors. This is just as true for large publicly traded vendors as it is for startups that provide essential materiel to the defense industry.

How the government addresses these risks in the future is up for debate and unclear. But one thing seems certain. Even if these kind of national security vendors may not be too big to fail, they may be too important to fail.

CHAPTER 15

THE FUTURE OF POLITICS

At the time this book was published, it wasn't certain how long the COVID-19 pandemic measures would remain in place, but one thing seems likely: As long as there are heightened concerns and precautions being taken, it will make voting difficult.

As we look ahead to the 2020 presidential election, the economy, COVID-19, national security, and other topics are likely to be very important in the debates. They will influence how people vote.

However, the way people vote will be most directly influenced by the question of whether COVID-19 remains a major concern or not. If COVID-19 concerns stretch out for a number of months going forward, we are likely to see a high number of people vote by absentee ballot.

Of course, it takes a lot more time to count absentee ballots. And this presents uncertainty and risks. In fact, the longer it takes to decide who wins elections, the more negative it is likely to be for business planning and financial markets.

How People Will Physically Vote

Voting by absentee ballot is not as instantaneous as when people vote electronically at polls, where their votes are counted on site immediately. Of course, there are faster ways to vote than by mailing in absentee ballots. And there are easier ways to vote remotely as well.

One example would be to do remote voting by text or using a computer login. Of course, there are many problems with this. The least of these problems is that some people do not own smartphones or computers. And whether you own a phone or computer should not be an issue to whether you can vote.

A much bigger problem, of course, is that switching over to an electronic voting system would be a very difficult thing — especially for a country as large as the United States. There would likely be a significant cost to creating and using this kind of system. Plus, we would need to see significant changes in approvals, including new permissions to record the data. And there would be challenges about data security and how voting records, systems, and counts would be protected. All of this increases the risk that we will be unable to get a remote electronic voting system up and running. In short, we are simply not prepared to handle it in the middle of a pandemic.

This is in stark contrast to the long-established use of absentee ballots and mail-in ballots. This doesn't require significant new technological platforms or new systems — although the volume would likely be at record levels.

Fortunately, absentee ballots are already something in place that have existed for some time. And they have been used in many different instances. In fact, since 1997, Texas residents can vote from outer space.[1]

It doesn't mean we shouldn't try to improve voting problems in the future — or that we shouldn't try to find a way to do this online. This is certainly worthy of discussion, but it takes time to get things done, and it would take a lot of budget. Something that does not take time is using a method to vote that already exists, and just expanding the number of people who use that method seems to be the best short-term stopgap solution — if one is required — in the 2020 U.S. election.

For more information about U.S. absentee ballots, check out the official website here:
https://www.usa.gov/absentee-voting#item-37337

In the long-term, the unique situation with COVID-19 may prompt a push toward online voting. And U.S. politicians may develop a means to remotely vote on congressional bills in the eventuality of similar kinds of future disruptions.

Determining Factor of the Presidential Election Outcome

The economy is likely to be the most critical issue for the 2020 presidential election — as it so often has been in the past. As I noted in my book *The Dumpster Fire Election*, as well as in my previous election book, *Midterm Economics*, the economy impacts the outcome of presidential elections.

Most important, is how the U.S. job market — and very specifically, changes in the unemployment rate — directly impact reelection campaigns.

Election Cyclicality

There is a historical relationship between the timing of presidential elections and the start of recessions over business cycles and elections since 1854.

In my analysis of election cyclicality, I have been most concerned with recession starts because the United States has been in its current business cycle expansion for a decade — since the Great Recession ended in June 2009. Our most recent business cycle has been the longest cycle in U.S. history.

But as I warned back in *The Dumpster Fire Election*, "this does not mean it will go on forever."

This is why it was important to assess the potential timing and start of the next recession. When targeting recession starts, I previously discovered a certain kind of *election cyclicality*, which has two main attributes related to how recessions and presidential elections coincide.

One attribute of election cyclicality is the election-recession window, which increases the odds of a recession starting shortly before or shortly after a U.S. presidential election.

This has held true for all but one recession since the Great Depression.

The second attribute is tied to a term limit on growth, which shows that there has never been a case of three full presidential terms without a recession starting.

This has held true since 1854, which is as far back as we have U.S. economic and recession data.

Election-Recession Windows

There is a narrow time frame in which recession starts happen, and this has often occurred around presidential elections. It's something I call the *election-recession window*.

If we look back to all of the official recessions since 1854, we find that the election-recession window has actually narrowed since 1928. In other words, since the Great Depression, recessions have started closer to elections than before. Plus, there has only been one recession start since 1928 that did not occur in the 11 months leading up to a presidential election or in the 13 months after a presidential election. This is a key part of the election-recession window — and we have been in it for months!

Term Limit on Growth

There are elections without recessions, but there have never been three consecutive presidential terms without a recession start. Never.

Since 1854, the historical maximum number of presidential terms without a recession start is two. There have been no exceptions. Think of it as a *term limit on growth*, which is the second attribute of election cyclicality.

As I noted in my June 2019 book *The Dumpster Fire Election*, "This means that if we consider all of U.S. business cycle history, we are likely to see the next recession start before the end of Trump's current term."

Based on what we are seeing now with the current and potential near-term economic impacts of COVID-19, the dynamics of election cyclicality and election-recession windows seem to be holding true.

The Importance of the Unemployment Rate

There have only been 12 one-term presidents in the history of the United States, with only three in the last hundred years: Carter, George H. W. Bush, and Hoover. In addition to these presidents, some people also consider Ford a one-term president since he replaced Nixon and ran for reelection — but he lost.

In all four of those instances — Carter, Bush, Hoover, and Ford — the U.S. unemployment rate was higher in the month before the presidential election than it had been during the November of the prior midterm election. This did not occur for any of the first terms of other U.S. presidents since 1930.

All of these increases, except for under Hoover, can be seen in Figure 15-1. The unemployment rate rose abysmally under Hoover during the Great Depression, from 3.2 percent at the end of 1930 (the year of the midterm election) to 16.9 percent by the end of 1932 (the year of the next presidential election).[2]

Figure 15-1: Economic Data Changes[3]

Economic Indicators	Midterm Election Year	Truman 1950	EH 1954	EH 2 1958	JFK/LBJ 1962	LBJ 1966	Nixon 1970	Nixon/Ford 1974	Carter 1978	Regan 1982	Regan 2 1986	BushM1 1990	Clinton 1994	Clinton 2 1998	Bush 43 2002	BushH43 2 2006	Obama 2010	Obama 2 2014
Housing Starts	Midterm Election Month (Nov)				1622	961	1647	1026	2094	1372	1623	1145	1511	1660	1753	1570	545	1001
	Month Before Next Pres Election (Oct)				1524	1569	2485	1629	1523	1590	1522	1244	1392	1549	2072	777	915	1327
	Change				-98	608	838	603	-571	218	-101	99	-119	-111	319	-793	370	326
Industrial Production	Midterm Election Month (Nov)	3.4	-0.1	0.7	1.1	2.5	-2.4	-2.5	3.3	-3.3	0.9	0.1	4.4	3.2	3.1	1.6	4.8	3.8
	Month Before Next Pres Election (Oct)	1.8	0.7	0.8	1.3	2.0	4.3	3.0	-1.7	2.9	1.9	1.9	3.8	2.4	3.2	-7.4	1.8	-1.3
	Change	-1.6	0.8	0.1	0.2	-0.5	6.7	5.5	-5.0	6.2	1.0	1.8	-0.6	-0.8	0.1	-9.0	-3.0	-5.1
Unemployment Rate	Midterm Election Month (Nov)	4.2	5.3	6.2	5.7	3.6	5.9	6.6	5.9	10.8	6.9	6.2	5.6	4.4	5.9	4.5	9.8	5.8
	Month Before Next Pres Election (Oct)	3.0	3.9	6.1	5.1	3.4	5.6	7.7	7.5	7.4	5.4	7.3	5.2	3.9	5.5	6.5	7.8	4.9
	Change	-1.2	-1.4	-0.1	-0.6	-0.2	-0.3	1.1	1.6	-3.4	-1.5	1.1	-0.4	-0.5	-0.4	2.0	-2.0	-0.9
Auto Sales	Midterm Election Month (Nov)								15.5	12.0	14.8	13.1	15.9	16.1	16.5	16.7	12.3	17.2
	Month Before Next Pres Election (Oct)								11.4	14.6	15.2	13.7	15.3	17.5	17.5	10.9	14.8	18.2
	Change								-4.1	2.6	0.4	0.6	-0.6	1.4	1.0	-5.8	2.5	1.0
Real GDP	Growth Rate in Midterm Year	8.7	-0.6	-0.7	6.1	6.6	0.2	-0.5	5.6	-1.9	3.5	1.9	4.0	4.4	1.8	2.7	2.5	2.6
	Growth Rate in Next Presidential Year	4.1	2.1	2.6	5.8	4.9	5.3	5.4	-0.2	7.3	4.2	3.6	3.8	4.1	3.8	-0.3	2.2	1.5
	Change	-4.6	2.7	3.3	-0.3	1.7	5.1	5.9	-5.8	9.2	0.7	1.6	-0.2	-0.4	2.0	-3.0	-0.3	-1.1

The Political Chessboard and Battleground States

As in 2020 — and most U.S. presidential elections — the geographic chessboard of electoral votes is set well ahead of the election, with battleground swing states holding critical sway over the outcome of the presidential election.

Of course, based on our analysis, the one thing that could potentially swing battleground states — and the election, in general — is the unemployment rate, as the data in Figure 15-1 implies with regards to second-term electability.

Implications for the 2020 Presidential Election

It makes sense that jobs matter. They always do! And the state of jobs and unemployment will likely matter in the 2020 election as well. In November 2018, the unemployment rate was 3.7 percent — near an all-time record low. But historic lows in the unemployment rate are difficult to maintain. Nevertheless, it seemed reasonable at even the beginning of 2020 to expect that the unemployment rate might still be low in October 2020.

However, the COVID-19 pandemic has flipped this expectation on its head, driving up the unemployment rate sharply, which is now likely to be well above the level seen in November 2018 by the time of the 2020 presidential election.

As a base case, I expect the impact of COVID-19 to be critical for the U.S. unemployment rate, which is likely to be exceptionally high in the second quarter of 2020. Furthermore, I expect elevated levels of unemployment and joblessness are likely to persist throughout 2020 and beyond.

In fact, based on the models I have built, it seems most likely that elevated unemployment rates may not return to pre-pandemic levels for at least two and a half years.

Based on the historical data of the past century regarding the U.S. unemployment rate and U.S. presidential elections, this would make the probability of a Trump reelection less likely.

Things That Change — and Things That Won't
Some things will change going into the 2020 presidential election — and some will remain the same. As you have seen in this chapter, the economy is important for how people vote — and that is likely to remain true in 2020.

Some big changes going into this election are likely to include greater bipartisan agreement on trade and supply chain risks, national security issues related to China, and the importance of deficit spending and the economy in the wake of COVID-19.

Of course, the candidates may differ greatly in their opinions as to what should have been done — and what will need to be done next — to stimulate the economy and help it recover. But the CARES Act had bipartisan support, and both parties are likely to leave fiscal conservatism in the past, as joblessness risks rise.

As I write this, the impact of COVID-19-induced weakness in the economy has yet to be fully seen. And given the unique situation we find ourselves in, historically considered, the outcome could also be quite unusual. Nevertheless, if the economy remains weak, it reduces the potential for President Trump's reelection.

CHAPTER 16

THE FUTURE OF LEADERSHIP

The future is going to be different than the present. And one of the most important things that's going to change is how people work.

The term for this continued (and potentially accelerating) set of changes is called "the future of work." As a leader, you need to know what's coming *and* what it means for projecting your leadership.

Not to cut to the punchline too quickly here, but the coming changes will make projecting leadership a much more important part of your job — especially if you want to climb an increasingly changing — and more geographically distributed corporate ladder.

One key trend that's been rapidly accelerating in recent years is remote work. In fact, between 2005 and 2015, the number of people working remotely more than doubled. And that pace shows no signs of slowing. In fact, it's likely to accelerate.

When I founded my financial research firm, Prestige Economics, in 2009, it was designed for remote work. We've never had an office. At the time some people thought I was crazy. Some people I know would have been less surprised if I told them I was going to join the circus.

But just 10 years later, in 2019, 30 percent of jobs were remote full time. And 54 percent of U.S. jobs entailed remote work at least once per month.[1]

That may sound like a lot, but it's still quite low from what I expect we'll see in the future.

Remote work is great. You might have more flexibility in how, when, and where you work. But you are also physically disconnected from your colleagues, your managers, and your customers. And the only way to bridge that gap is to do something impactful — to do something visible.

Doing a good job is important. That's always mission #1. But it's really not enough — especially if you want to rise above a field of increasingly dispersed workers.

You've heard people say, "You need to stand out to be outstanding"? Well, that's the key!

You need a positive way to stand out. You need to project what you know to reach people separated by space and time — or at least maybe a few time zones.

Building your visibility as a leader is not just an exercise for the present. And as you can see, it will actually become an increasingly necessary ingredient for success and advancement in the future.

This is perhaps one of the greatest professional realizations that is likely to come as a result of the experience of remote work in the face of the COVID-19 pandemic.

That you need to be able to effectively project leadership remotely.

CHAPTER 17

THE FUTURE OF TRAVEL AND LEISURE

The travel and leisure industries have been devastated by COVID-19. And there are likely to be impacts on travel and leisure throughout the year — and potentially well into the future.

This all begins with a question: How quickly after COVID-19 passes will you be willing to travel to Vegas and go to a casino — or go to Orlando and visit a theme park?

This is the kind of question that will drastically impact travel in the coming year or two. But as we look beyond this year, we have to think about how the future of travel and leisure may be impacted as a long-term result of COVID-19.

What kind of impacts do we expect for the means of travel, the destinations, and the potential for new trends that could arise from this unique situation?

Let's dig in!

Risks to Tourist Centers and Related Businesses

Some of the biggest negative risks and impacts from COVID-19 this year and next year are likely to be on major tourist centers, like Las Vegas, Orlando, and New Orleans.

And the negative impacts could have significant economic shockwaves for other cities with a lot of other tourism and conference demand, like New York City, Austin, Houston, San Diego, Asheville, and many others.

This loss of business is likely to directly impact the workers and companies in the tourism industry. But it is also likely to impact other industries as a second-order impact. And there may even be negative third-order impacts.

In fact, reduced travel and conference demand could be far reaching, with potentially deleterious impacts on regional housing markets tied to tourism centers.

Part of these negative economic risks stem from government regulations to avoid crowds, but there is also likely to be a reduction in disposable income that could also have negative impacts on tourism and tourist centers in the year ahead — and beyond.

Impacts of a Forced Staycation

While near-term downside risks to tourism centers seem highly likely, the medium-term impact on tourism of the COVID-19 experience is a bit more mixed — and uncertain.

There are questions that will determine how this plays out.

For example, what if people generally enjoyed having a forced staycation of sorts as a result of the COVID-19 "shelter in place" requirements?

After all, if they did, it may mean that in the future — based on the positive experience of having had a mandated staycation — some people may actually prefer them over vacations with travel to exotic places.

This is not a guarantee or a hypothesis.

This is just a potential future outcome.

Whenever people have a new experience, there is a chance that some might like it. Of course, some may hate it.

Yes, some people might prefer staycations in the future. This notion is still a relatively new one, and the use of the word only came into use less than 20 years ago. Since then, there's been a trend around staycations.

I've taken them, and I find them quite enjoyable.

But just as some people may find that they enjoyed their forced staycations, some will no doubt hate it. In fact, we may see that other people decide — as a direct result of this experience — that they never want to spend so much time in their homes again.

Such an experience could actually engender increased travel and vacation demand over time.

Whether people will have generally enjoyed or hated their forced staycations will impact future travel demand in the medium term. And their experience is still up for debate.

No matter the experience, one thing does seem certain, though: People are likely to be more cognizant of social distance in the future — for both the near term and the medium term.

Only in the long term do these impacts seem likely to be potentially reversed.

In the near term, this means that festivals, theme parks, crowded resorts, carnivals, fairs, concerts, and other large gatherings may be things that people eschew when they go on vacation.

So even if people go away on vacation this summer or this year, they are likely to go somewhere that is less crowded with just a bit more distance.

Of course, this is unlikely to be true for *all* people. But we aren't considering individual travel decisions. We need to consider decisions at the population level. So, even if some people continue undisturbed by the impact of COVID-19, we need to consider that it seems much more likely that the population as a whole might change its behavior — at least in the immediate term, when COVID-19 fears, social distancing norms, and financial concerns are most prominent.

Long-Term COVID-19 Risks

In addition to dynamics that impact travel in general, we may also find that there are some cities that suffer for years with bouts of COVID-19 flowing in and out of various areas at different times. Essentially, this risk could result in what become essentially rolling travel brownouts of activity, as "shelter in place" orders, travel bans, and quarantines pop up across different regions.

Next month, it could be New York.

The month after, it might be Los Angeles.

And yet the month after that, it could be Miami or Chicago.

As with the impact of staycations, the potential for rolling travel bans or COVID-19 hot spot policies seem less certain. This seems especially true compared to the more certain expectation that a lot more people will work remotely in the future — or saying that we might see changes in the way people perceive online education as a result of forced at-home, in-hand education in a COVID-19 world.

Dynamics Likely to Be True

For some travel topics, this is an area where the future simply cannot be as clear, and we need to consider various alternative futures.

But there are a couple things that seem very likely to be true when it comes to travel and leisure.

First, travel and leisure are generally funded by disposable income. This is true for individuals, and it is also true at the corporate level. This means that both personal and business funds for travel and leisure are likely to fall if the economy remains under pressure.

Corporate travel departments clamp down hard and fast when cash flow slows. This means that even if the conference business could come back as COVID-19 fears and risks fade, companies may be slow to spend the money for conferences without direct ROI.

It could be especially grim for the travel industry if people don't get their jobs back in those industries. But even if workers in travel, tourism, and leisure get their jobs back, travel companies, like airlines, could see their profit margins fall — even after travel ramps back up.

After all, airlines make their best margins on last-minute business travelers, as well as on business class and first class seats. This is why when demand for business travel falls, so does the profitability of airlines.

The profitable business conference industry could also suffer as well. And this would have a negative impact on hotels.

Overall, people and companies are less likely to spend money on something that is not a necessity like leisure and travel, at least in the coming year or two or so.

Business class seats on international flights are also usually extremely profitable as well, which is why airlines compete so much for those long-haul routes. But tighter travel policies reduce demand for business class seats — as does a big drop in perceived individual wealth that accompanies a significant drop in equity markets, like the ones we have so recently seen.

Of course, expecting international flights to be restored in the immediate term would be very optimistic.

Risks for International Travel
International travel could remain very difficult — if not impossible — as a result of the COVID-19 pandemic.

In recent discussions with executives, we've debated at what point in time it might be safe to plan an international trip. By that, our discussion has focused on identifying what time one might be able to take a trip to Europe, for example.

The question here is, when could you plan a two-week trip to Europe that only takes two weeks — and not six weeks?

In other words, when would a European trip not require a two-week mandatory quarantine when you get there, and then require another two-week quarantine when you get back.

That might take months — or it might take much longer.

That kind of travel agenda is just not efficient.

And that's going to be a problem for companies trying to do business that requires in-person international travel.

The truth is that not only might it take months — or longer — before international travel is "normal" again. But in the future, it seems likely that international flight travel bans may be much more quickly implemented than they were during the COVID-19 outbreak.

Downside Cruise Line Risks

Cruise lines seem likely to experience significant financial and business problems going forward. The risks are underscored by the outbreak on the *Diamond Princess*, which was one of the first flashpoints of COVID-19.

Historically, whenever there have been various disease outbreaks, cruise lines tend to get caught in the middle of it. In general, cruises are the highest-value form of travel. After all, you get to go to numerous destinations, and the food is included.

All in all, the value of cruising is exceptionally high. This is one of the reasons it's become so popular in recent years. However, you do put people quite literally in closer quarters. And those close quarters become a greater risk in a pandemic-type scenario, which is what happened on the *Diamond Princess* at the beginning of the coronavirus outbreak.

Looking ahead for this year, next year, and potentially for several years beyond, we expect there might be significantly reduced demand for cruises.

This drop in demand wouldn't just stem from a drop in disposable income, but it may also be a function of aggregate demand reduction at the population level, stemming from COVID-19 concerns and elevated social distancing norms.

Long-Term Professional Changes
There is another potential significant travel impact that could happen as a result of COVID-19. It seems likely that some people may opt to completely change their careers and business travel as a result of their experience following the outbreak of COVID-19.

In short, forced reductions of travel may lead some business travelers to change their careers, jobs, and lives to necessitate less travel.

I know this has been the case with my own life in which I'm normally on the road almost nonstop. But as a result of the COVID-19 pandemic, I've been forced to change how I conduct business.

If that were to be something I continue to do, it could drastically reduce my own travel. And if this occurs at the aggregate travel, total overall travel demand may decline at the population level.

If higher-margin business travelers fly less overall, this could result in reduced aggregate miles flown demand. And it could reduce the number of profitable corporate miles flow.

We may also see that in the same way that people increase their remote working and telecommuting as a result of the COVID-19 pandemic, they may also increase the amount of remote conferencing and remote meetings they do, rather than doing as many in-person meetings as they had in the past.

This isn't necessarily just a cost-reducing thing right?

It is also like the impact of commuting less. Because when you spend less time commuting, you spend less money on gasoline, and it saves you money. But more importantly, it saves you time — and that's especially true when we think about flying places for meetings.

It is not so much the plane ticket that's the greatest cost.

It's the hours of travel time both ways and the stress of business travel that comprises the greatest cost people might be trying to avoid.

I know you might be reading this and thinking, "I love travel so much." But business travel is honestly a completely separate animal — and most businesspeople refer to business travel simply as *the road.*

And let me tell you, the road is a grind.

The Future of Travel and Leisure

In sum, we're going to see some significant changes in the way people travel in the future. The most significant changes are probably going to be in the more near term, when there is significantly reduced demand for travel and leisure across sectors that stems from a mix of an overhang of social distancing norms and COVID-19 fears, as well as disposable income reductions and a drop in corporate business expenditures.

Personal space is not something you find in great abundance in most airplanes. And because of an overhang in new social distancing norms and COVID-19 fears, I expect that we may find that reduced flight demand persists for a significant and protracted period of time, even though there might be a certain segment of the population that just can't wait to go somewhere.

In the long run, we could see a societal shift in the way people perceive travel, and this seems likely to have a potentially negative impact for travel companies.

Now, there is one counterpoint for this, and that would be related to people who have a real *Wanderlust* right now. People who are locked up in condos — especially in population-dense, heavily urban areas — may be crawling for the walls and dying to just get out there and travel anywhere.

That may be true, but those would-be travelers could likely find many of their destinations are not immediately serviceable by flights. As such, they may end up on road trips in the near term rather than flying places. But there will always be places to go.

CHAPTER 18

THE FUTURE OF ESG AND SUSTAINABILITY

The COVID-19 pandemic has the potential to impact ESG and sustainability activist investor initiatives and long-term corporate strategic planning.

Some of the most important data people have been looking at to gauge the impact and timing of a COVID-19 pandemic has been Chinese emissions, specifically nitrogen dioxide.

With the initial outbreak of the COVID-19 coronavirus in Wuhan, China implemented a massive quarantine — and Chinese manufacturing all but ceased, as did Chinese emissions.

I mention this topic because ESG activist investor demands have been sharply on the rise. In 2018, there were record levels of activist investor demands, both in the United States and globally. This can be seen in Figure 18-2 and Figure 18-1, respectively.

Plus, in 2018, some of the top areas where there were activist investors pushing for goals and initiatives included climate change (19%), sustainability (13%), other environmental (7%), and political activity (19%).[1] You can see the breakdown in Figure 18-3. If we consider sustainability a type of environmental initiative along with climate change and other environmental resolutions, we see that 39% — a plurality — of all activist investor resolutions filed in 2018 were environment related.

I want to be careful here on one point. I am not putting a value judgement on these resolutions. I merely wish to show that they were a plurality of activist investor resolutions in 2018 — and that they are likely to become increasingly common.

And they will become increasingly important in finance.

In short, activist investors are usually large investors that use their shareholder power to push companies to make fundamental changes in the way they operate.

And their activities have been on the rise. In fact, the number of companies subject to activist demands globally rose by almost 54 percent between 2013 and 2018. This can be seen in Figure 18-1.

Domestically, the situation is very similar, and the number of U.S. companies subject to activist demands is up by over 50 percent since 2013. This can be seen in Figure 18-2.

Figure 18-1: Global Companies Subject to Activist Demands[2]

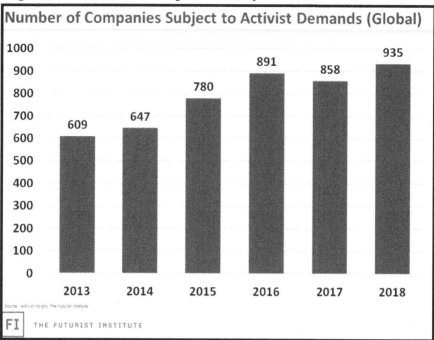

Figure 18-2: U.S. Companies Subject to Activist Demands[3]

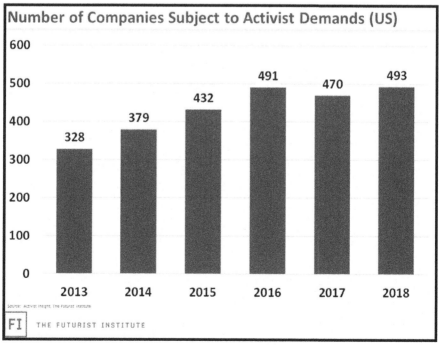

Looking at the future of finance, I expect that this dynamic of rising activist demands — and the number of companies impacted — is likely to continue rising on trend.

Any undergraduate economics student knows that companies often benefit from things they don't pay for but that have costs. These costs that are not captured but are passed on to society at large are called externalities. These include any potentially negative environmental impact a business's operations have. But they can also involve leveraging certain labor, societal, or political inefficiencies to capture an arbitrage opportunity to reap outsized financial benefits.

Figure 18-3: Type of Activist Resolutions Filed in 2018[4]

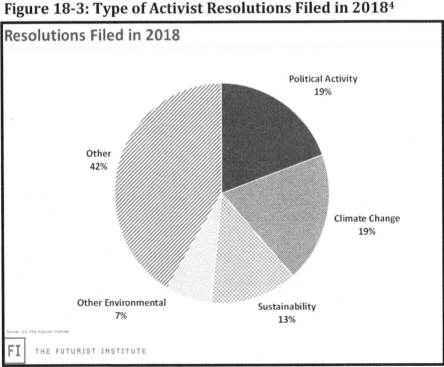

Resolutions Filed in 2018

Political Activity 19%

Climate Change 19%

Sustainability 13%

Other Environmental 7%

Other 42%

Source: S2, The Futurist Institute

FI THE FUTURIST INSTITUTE

It should therefore not be a surprise that there has been a push to hold companies responsible for these externalities. After all, this is one of the very first things most economics students learn.

But here's the deal: Fully pricing in externalities to company operations is likely to erode profitability for some companies. And that may be just the beginning. Ratings agencies have already started warning companies I work with in the energy space that their sustainability goals (or lack thereof) could impact their bond prices and their weighted average cost of capital — their WACC.[5] This could in turn impact their profitability, overall valuation, credit rating, and equity prices.

Looking Ahead

In the future, companies will increasingly need to demonstrate achievable sustainability and other ESG goals. If they don't, they will be at the mercy of activist investors. And their profitability and share prices may very well suffer.

Furthermore, reduced emissions from shut-in manufacturing capacity, remote work, remote schooling, and reduced travel could inspire activist investors to support adopting some of these now necessary changes permanently once the COVID-19 pandemic crisis has passed.

The logic for this kind of push to adopt these extraordinary actions stems from a belief that if a company wants to show it is greener, what better way is there to do that than by:
— Reducing commuter fuel consumption of the office staff.
— Reducing power consumption in the office.
— Reducing jet fuel demand and the CO_2 footprint that accompanies extensive (and especially international) business travel.

It is my expectation that some companies may carry the experience and policies of reduced energy consumption forward. And for some activist investors, this experience is likely to reveal that carbon emissions can be cut significantly if a tremendous commitment to that endeavor is made.

But even if companies were to fully return to operating their businesses exactly as they had before the COVID-19 pandemic outbreak, I would still expect the number of activist investor initiatives to increase on trend over time. And I would still expect sustainability and climate change to remain at the top of the shortlist no matter what.

As in other areas, the COVID-19 pandemic has revealed for ESG and sustainability a potential that already existed but was not being acted on. In this case, the potential revealed was the potential to materially reduce energy consumption and emissions.

CHAPTER 19

THE FUTURE OF STARTUPS

Startup culture has exploded during the most recent business cycle. But now, because of the COVID-19 pandemic, the future of startup life is at risk.

The problems and risks stem from how startups are funded, the way they operate at losses, and their relatively small size.

First, startups are generally funded privately, usually by wealthy investors, known as *angel investors*. But even wealthy investors are impacted by declines in equity markets and increased financial market risks — in fact, they are likely to be much more sensitive to market moves than the average person. So, with the recent drop in the stock market and economic uncertainty ahead, private funding is likely to slow for many investments.

Beyond a risk of funding loss as a knock-on effect from dynamics in other markets, there is also the potential for investors to change their rubric of investing in these more uncertain times. And that could be a problem for startups that try to grow fast.

There have been countless jokes — including the lampooning of startup life on the TV show *Silicon Valley* — about how the more startups lose, the more they are worth. Having been an angel investor, as well as a brief stint as an executive at a FinTech startup, I can say that this dynamic and mindset is absolutely pervasive, irresponsible, and infuriating.

To anyone with a finance background, this notion feels really upside down. But it isn't just something that's been plaguing private money deals. After all, you can see there is some truth to the notion of being more valuable the more you lose; if we look at the IPO data in "The Future of Finance" chapter, this doesn't seem hard to believe.

At times like these, investors in public markets often look for cash on a corporate balance sheet and positive cash flow as signals of health and value. But many startups are the opposite of that. This means that running negative cash flow and net losses is now about to be unsustainable.

It's a business model about to go the way of the dodo. And with a change in priorities from growth to cash flow, it means startup life — as it existed for the second half of the last decade — is in big trouble.

To top off the risks that the money well is about to run dry, and companies that increase their value by losing money are about to find their business model reevaluated, it's important to consider that many startups will likely not be qualified to receive the same kind of CARES Act bailout funds as other companies.

Because many startups survive only by fundraised check to fundraised check, many of them are very unlikely to qualify for the forgivable SBA loan bailouts that are part of the $2.3 trillion CARES Act.

In other words, the money is about to run out. And not even a government bailout can help most companies that operate like this.

Of course, there will be exceptions.

Startups in MedTech, EdTech, e-commerce, and national security have the greatest chance of making it through this disruptive period. Their ability to provide critical solutions at a time like this could still draw in capital.

But even they will need to make payroll.

And, unfortunately, not all of them will. So, even some critical startups may fail.

Impacts and Expectations

For at least the next year or so, startups are likely to have a very tougher time raising funds — especially if they run with big losses and have little or no cash flow. This could kill countless startups and decimate entire startup ecosystems, like the one in my city of Austin.

But the impacts could be felt throughout the coming decade.

If we look beyond this business cycle, it seems likely that the future of startups may be more austere for some time to come.

And that may not be a bad thing.

From a business standpoint, you want companies that make money to grow. And choosing growth over profits is always a tough trade-off. But in the future, profits and cash flow may be prioritized over growth.

Of course, this could hinder the pace of some innovations, which would be a negative impact. And one that may have great cost. But these changes in priorities could also result in more sound financial business models.

In the near term and for many years to come, startups will need to be — and show that they are — more financially sound.

Even after the COVID-19 pandemic passes, public equity markets rise, and growth returns, we are likely to find that businesses that lose money will lose out to those that can rapidly show positive profits.

It should have always been this way, and now it is more likely to be.

CHAPTER 20

THE FUTURE OF RECESSION

I'm an economist today because I got caught in the 2001 recession.

I wasn't an economist, and my ignorance of the economy put me in a bad place.

Now, almost 20 years later, I'm an economist and a financial futurist. I spend almost every minute of my working life analyzing the financial systems around us as well as analyzing dynamics that could shape our world in the long run.

As I think about the 20-year shadow that recession in 2001 cast on my life, I have begun to think about the shadow that the 2020 recession and the COVID-19 experience is likely to cast forward over the next 20 years. I expect that the experience of the COVID-19 pandemic will inspire more people to go into recession-proof industries, like healthcare.

But before I get too deep into the punchline, let me share my story with you.

The Second Dumbest Thought I Ever Had

It was a sunny spring day in 1999, and I had just gotten out of an economics class at the University of Virginia. There I was, standing in the sunshine on The Lawn of these beautiful historic Grounds, and everything seemed right in the universe. I was finishing up my undergrad, and I had an offer to pursue a Master's in German at the University of North Carolina, Chapel Hill.

It was a full ride — tuition, health insurance, living allowance, everything. It was tremendous funding for a graduate student. On top of that, all of my friends in similar degree programs were landing six-figure consulting jobs right out of college. It was the era of the supercharged dot-com boom — the best job market in the history of the United States. I knew I could easily score a good job in the private sector if I wanted it.

I was spoiled with two great options, and I wasn't sure which to go for. I liked being a student, and I wanted to learn more, so I figured that I'd go for the grad school option. After all, *if the economy is rocking now, just think how great it will be in a few more years! And by then I'll have a Master's degree, so I'll make even* more *money!*

That was the second dumbest thought I ever had. I wasn't thinking like an economist. I wasn't thinking about the business cycle, the inevitability of bad times following good. I wasn't thinking about the way that the economy can kick you in the ass.

Of course, I wasn't yet an economist.

So I signed up for grad school, I got my Master's, and I reentered the job market in the spring of 2001. Oh, what a difference two years makes!

The same companies that were offering $10,000, $15,000, or $25,000 signing bonuses in the fall of 2000 were now shedding employees like they were going out of style.

I met people who had received written job offers in 1999 or 2000, and then the companies deferred them for a year or two. A number of those deferrals became permanent, as many people never, ever received those jobs.

If it's good now, it'll be even better tomorrow!

That's the second dumbest thought I ever had. It's a lesson I learned before I became a business economist, and it's the most important thing about the economy that I share with people who are not economists.

The very dumbest thought I ever had was "That bull ain't gonna turn around."

That happened on July 12, 1997 in Pamplona, Spain. But that's a story for another day.

When it comes to surviving and thriving in a recession, there are some thoughts that a lot of people have that are just as dumb as the belief *that bull ain't gonna turn around.*

I already shared one of those thoughts:

"If the economy is rocking now, just think how great it will be in a few more years!"

And here are a few others:

"I don't need to build a network outside of the company where I work. There will always be work for me here at ABC Industries."

"I'm an expert in my job. Why should I get more training? No one could ever replace me."

"My company is laying people off left, right, and center, but that's okay. I'm indispensable. I'll just hunker down at my company and wait for the recession to pass."

The sad truth is, people with these kinds of attitudes — and many people have these kinds of attitudes, even if they don't realize it themselves — are probably not going to be okay in the coming economic downturn.

In all likelihood, they are going to get gored.

Having options is the name of the game. Recessions take options away, and you need to find way to create new options. You can minimize the damage personally and professionally.

You may even use a recession as an opportunity, as I did—as a chance to change your career, get more education, become more valuable for your company, or start a business.

Thinking About the 20-Year Shadow of COVID-19

If we think about recessions and career planning, it is important to consider that people will want to create more options for themselves.

The long-term impact of the 2001 recession on my professional development is something we may see again. And as a result of COVID-19 — and a potential ensuing recession — we are likely to see an entire generation of young people watch this unfold and make decisions to create options.

While I became an economist after the 2001 tech bubble, the nature of COVID-19 and a recession that stems from it seems likely to inspire more people to go into healthcare or to get remote jobs — or at least jobs that could be remote.

Future Recessions

We are likely to see recessions continue to occur in the future. After all, the economy is called a business cycle for a reason.

CHAPTER 21

WEIGHING IMPACTS

The human tragedy of the COVID-19 pandemic is likely to be massive. The loss of life, illness, human impact, and economic damage of the COVID-19 pandemic is likely to be beyond catastrophic.

The near-term negative impacts for entire industries and segments of the economy could be significantly detrimental for years to come. But there is the potential that out of this crisis and tragedy some long-term upside potential for public health, the economy, and society overall may yet be achievable.

Of course, as we look for the upside in these dark times, it is important to realize that the medical, economic, social, and personal benefits of not having this pandemic would obviously be the best-case scenario overall.

But that is not reality.

We are in a pandemic.

The Future Potential Impacts

With the losses, risks, and costs in mind, we should consider that the potential future impacts of the COVID-19 pandemic could have some positive impacts.

Increased remote work can materially impact the way people work and live. It's been a growing trend for some time, but the COVID-19 pandemic is a threshold moment that could push remote work sharply forward.

Increased access to online education can materially impact people's professional and working lives, including the professional and career options they have, as well as the potential future incomes they earn. Postsecondary educational attainment, including degree and certification completion, are likely to increase. Plus, there is likely to be an increase in the number of home-schooled pupils, which could result in better outcomes for some learners who had not previously considered home schooling or online education.

Increased healthcare prioritization is also likely. Choices in education, investments, and policies may lead to improved overall public health outcomes. The number of people studying medical and healthcare subjects is likely to increase. And the medical supply chain in the United States is likely to be shored up and secured to reduce the likelihood of medical device and PPE shortages in the future. Additionally, we may find individuals become more aware of their own personal health as a result of the COVID-19 pandemic. This could have a long-term impact.

Lower energy consumption and emissions also seem likely for a time, as an economic slowdown, remote work, and social distancing norms reduce petroleum fuels consumption. And that, too, could have a longer-term impact in how companies view and implement sustainability strategies.

On the downside, countless industries will never be the same, including tourism and leisure industries. They are likely to feel revenue-sapping aftershocks from the COVID-19 pandemic for years to come. And there may be long-term impacts on travel and leisure industries from new societal norms of social distancing.

Of course, the greatest negative impacts in the long run are likely to be further leaning in to deficit spending and running up an ever-greater national debt. And there is the growing risk that we are asymptotically approaching a future quantum state of the economy in which the Fed owns everything with nothing at the same time.

Yet, there is the potential for some positive impacts to be found in this watershed moment for public health, education, and the economy.

But the price we will have paid in the end for the benefits derived from the COVID-19 pandemic will be far too high. And that will be true in terms of lost lives, human suffering, a strained healthcare system, regional and industry economic devastation, a rise in the national debt, and greater central bank obligations.

THE FUTURE AFTER COVID

My main goal in writing this book was to share my views of the potential future dynamics that could result and have long-term impacts as a result of the COVID-19 pandemic.

I have laid out some of the most likely scenarios for potential COVID-19 impacts. And I have also tried to focus on some of the most important as-yet-unanswered questions that will have long-lived impacts. Of course, the COVID-19 situation is rapidly evolving, and many of the issues in this book may change drastically — or reach some level of resolution — more quickly than anticipated, depending on those developments.

One thing seems certain, however: Many industries, businesses, individuals, and economies will be seriously impacted — both negatively and positively. There are opportunities for long-run positive impacts in the way we work, access education, prioritize the strength of our supply chain, improve access to food and paper products, and secure the future quality of (and access to) healthcare we experience. But the costs will be high.

The future is uncertain, so it is critical to look for long-term trends with the greatest potential to persist in many different alternative futures scenarios. And it is important to consider the risk factors and levers of change that could challenge your assumptions of the future.

I hope this book helped you achieve those ends.

Further Learning

If you've enjoyed this book and want to learn more about planning strategically for an uncertain future as well as alternative futures, I recommend pursuing the Certified Futurist and Long-Term Analyst™ — FLTA™ — training program that I created for The Futurist Institute. The goal of this certification is to help analysts, executives, and professionals incorporate new and emerging trends and technologies into long-term strategic planning.

The FLTA™ certification program has six distinct professional tracks, including consulting, national security, financial planning, accounting, legal, and standard tracks. Plus, The Futurist Institute is accredited by the Certified Financial Planner Board of Standards® as a provider of continuing education hours. And the FLTA program includes 8.5 hours of CFP® continuing education. It is also eligible for continuing education hours from other organizations as well.

All of the details about the FLTA™ and The Futurist Institute can be found at www.futuristinstitute.org.

Your Next Steps

For now, the most important thing is to try and keep yourself and your loved ones out of harm's way. The importance of social distancing has been stressed repeatedly by healthcare professionals and public health policy leaders.

This crisis, too, shall pass.

And when it does, planning for the long-term potential impacts will be critical. This includes accepting that some of the short-term adaptations implemented during the time of the COVID-19 pandemic may be permanent.

And preparing for second-order and third-order financial market and economic fallout will be critical.

Recovery will come. And if you look for opportunities to help your organization improve — or if you find ways to adapt and reshape your career — in the wake of this tragedy, you may be able to hasten the speed of that recovery.

Good luck and be well!

~ Jason Schenker
April 2020

ENDNOTES

Chapter 3
1. Bureau of Labor Statistics. Retrieved on 2 April 2020 from https://www.bls.gov/ooh/most-new-jobs.htm
2. Bureau of Labor Statistics: Retrieved on 2 April 2020 from https://www.bls.gov/ooh/fastest-growing.htm
3. NBER, FRED, World Bank, Prestige Economics. Retrieved February 17, 2017:
http://www.nber.org/chapters/c1567.pdf
https://fraser.stlouisfed.org/files/docs/publications/frbslreview/rev_stls_198706.pdf
http://databank.worldbank.org/data/reports.aspx?source=world-development-indicators#
4. U.S. Bureau of Labor Statistics, All Employees, Warehousing and Storage [CES4349300001], retrieved from FRED, Federal Reserve Bank of St. Louis; https://fred.stlouisfed.org/series/CES4349300001, April 1, 2020.

Chapter 4
1. U.S. Bureau of Labor Statistics, Consumer Price Index for All Urban Consumers: All Items in U.S. City Average [CPIAUCSL], retrieved from FRED, Federal Reserve Bank of St. Louis; https://fred.stlouisfed.org/series/CPIAUCSL, April 1, 2020.
U.S. Bureau of Labor Statistics, Consumer Price Index for All Urban Consumers: Medical Care in U.S. City Average [CPIMEDSL], retrieved from FRED, Federal Reserve Bank of St. Louis; https://fred.stlouisfed.org/series/CPIMEDSL, April 1, 2020.
2. Ibid.
3. Department of Education. Retrieved on 2 April 2020. https://nces.ed.gov/programs/digest/d18/tables/dt18_206.10.asp
4. Ibid.
5. Bureau of Labor Statistics. Retrieved on 2 April 2020 from https://www.bls.gov/emp/graphics/2019/unemployment-rates-and-earnings.htm

Chapter 5
1. "2017 State of Telecommuting in the U.S. Employee Workforce." Flexjobs. Retrieved on 9 May 2019 from https://www.flexjobs.com/2017-State-of-Telecommuting-US.
2. Ibid.

Chapter 6
1. Ritter, Jay R. (9 April 2019). "IPO Data." *Warrington College of Business*, University of Florida. Retrieved on 2 April 2020 from site.warrington.ufl.edu/ritter/ipo-data/.
2. Ibid.
3. Ibid.
4. Ibid.
5. "Household Debt and Credit." New York Federal Reserve Bank. Retrieved on 2 April 2020 from https://www.newyorkfed.org/medialibrary/interactives/householdcredit/data/pdf/HHDC_2019Q4.pdf
6. Ibid.

Chapter 7
1. Federal Reserve. "The Federal Reserve's Monetary Policy Toolkit: Past, Present, and Future." Retrieved from https://www.federalreserve.gov/newsevents/speech/yellen20160826a.htm
2. Board of Governors of the Federal Reserve System (US), Assets: Total Assets: Total Assets (Less Eliminations From Consolidation): Wednesday Level [WALCL], retrieved from FRED, Federal Reserve Bank of St. Louis; https://fred.stlouisfed.org/series/WALCL, April 1, 2020.

Chapter 8

1. Committee for a Responsible Federal Budget. "What's in the $2 Trillion Coronavirus Relief Package?" Retrieved on 2 April 2020 from http://www.crfb.org/blogs/whats-2-trillion-coronavirus-relief-package.
2. Bureau of Economic Analysis. "Gross Domestic Product , Fourth Quarter and Year 2019." Retrieved on 2 April 2020 from https://www.bea.gov/system/files/2020-02/gdp4q19_2nd_0.pdf.
3. U.S. Department of the Treasury. Fiscal Service, Federal Debt: Total Public Debt [GFDEBTN], retrieved from FRED, Federal Reserve Bank of St. Louis; https://fred.stlouisfed.org/series/GFDEBTN, April 1, 2020.
4. Ibid.
5. Federal Reserve Bank of St. Louis and U.S. Office of Management and Budget, Federal Debt: Total Public Debt as Percent of Gross Domestic Product [GFDEGDQ188S], retrieved from FRED, Federal Reserve Bank of St. Louis; https://fred.stlouisfed.org/series/GFDEGDQ188S, April 1, 2020.
6. Desjardins, J. (6 August 2015). "$60 Trillion of World Debt in One Visualization." Visual Capitalist. Retrieved 11 February 2017: http://www.visualcapitalist.com/60-trillion-of-world-debt-in-one-visualization/.
7. Mayer, J. (18 November 2015). "The Social Security Façade." Retrieved 11 February 2017: http://www.usnews.com/opinion/economic-intelligence/2015/11/18/social-security-and-medicare-have-morphed-into-unsustainable-entitlements.
8. U.S. Social Security Administration. "Social Security History: Otto von Bismarck." Sourced from https://www.ssa.gov/history/ottob.html.
9. Image provided courtesy of The Heritage Foundation. Retrieved 11 February 2017: http://thf_media.s3.amazonaws.com/infographics/2014/10/BG-eliminate-waste-control-spending-chart-3_HIGHRES.jpg.
10. Twarog, S. (January 1997). "Heights and Living Standards in Germany, 1850-1939: The Case of Wurttemberg" as reprinted in *Health and Welfare During Industrialization.* Steckel, R. and F. Roderick, eds. Chicago: University of Chicago Press, p. 315. Retrieved 11 February 2017: http://www.nber.org/chapters/c7434.pdf.
11. U.S. Social Security Administration. "Social Security History: Otto von Bismarck." Sourced from https://www.ssa.gov/history/ottob.html.
12. U.S. Social Security Administration. *Fast Facts and Figures About Social Security, 2017*, p. 8. Retrieved on 17 June 2019: https://www.ssa.gov/policy/docs/chartbooks/fast_facts/.
13. World Bank, Population Growth for the United States [SPPOPGROWUSA], retrieved from FRED, Federal Reserve Bank of St. Louis; https://fred.stlouisfed.org/series/SPPOPGROWUSA, June 5, 2018.
14. Last, J. (2013) *What to Expect, When No One's Expecting: America's Coming Demographic Disaster.* New York: Encounter Books, pp. 2-4.
15. Ibid., p. 3.
16. Last (2013), p. 109.
17. U.S. Social Security Administration. Retrieved 11 February 2017 from https://www.ssa.gov/history/ratios.html Last (2013) also uses a similar table in his book on p. 108.
18. Last (2013), p. 107.

Chapter 13

1. This is an allusion to Graham Allison's book *Destined for War: Can America and China Escape Thucydides's Trap?* (2017).

Chapter 15

1. "The First American to Vote from Space." (8 November 2016). *The Atlantic.* https://www.theatlantic.com/science/archive/2016/11/voting-from-space/506960/
2. U.S. Bureau of Labor Statistics, Unemployment Rate [UNRATE], retrieved from FRED, Federal Reserve Bank of St. Louis; https://fred.stlouisfed.org/series/UNRATE, April 1, 2020.
3. Ibid.

Chapter 16
1.Retrieved on 12 January 2020 from https://www.owllabs.com/state-of-remote-work/2019

Chapter 18
1. Welsh, H. (9 November 2018). "Social, Environmental & Sustainable Governance Shareholder Proposals in 2018." *Securities and Exchange Commission*, Sustainable Investments Institute. Retrieved on 12 July 2019 from www.sec.gov/comments/4-725/4725-4636528-176443.pdf.
2. "Shareholder Activism in Q1 2019." (April 2019). *Reports*. Activist Insight. Retrieved on 12 July 2019 from www.activistinsight.com/research/ShareholderActivism_Q12019.pdf.
3. Ibid.
4. Welsh, H. (9 November 2018). "Social, Environmental & Sustainable Governance Shareholder Proposals in 2018." *Securities and Exchange Commission*, Sustainable Investments Institute. Retrieved on 12 July 2019 from www.sec.gov/comments/4-725/4725-4636528-176443.pdf. of ESG oversight.
5."Exxon Board Targeted for Lack of ESG Oversight." (May 11, 2019). National Association of Corporate Directors. Retrieved on 12 July 2019 https://tinyurl.com/NACDExxon2019.

ABOUT THE AUTHOR

Mr. Schenker is the President of Prestige Economics and Chairman of The Futurist Institute. He has been ranked one of the most accurate financial forecasters and futurists in the world. Bloomberg News has ranked Mr. Schenker a top forecaster in 43 categories, including #1 in the world for his accuracy in 25 categories, including for his forecasts of the Euro, the British Pound, the Russian Ruble, the Chinese RMB, crude oil prices, natural gas prices, gold prices, industrial metals prices, agricultural commodity prices, and U.S. jobs.

Mr. Schenker was ranked one of the top 100 most influential financial advisors in the world by Investopedia in 2018. His work has been featured in *The Wall Street Journal*, *The New York Times*, and the *Frankfurter Allgemeine Zeitung*. He has appeared on CNBC, CNN, ABC, NBC, MSNBC, Fox, Fox Business, BNN, Bloomberg Germany, and the BBC. Mr. Schenker has been a guest host of Bloomberg Television and he is a columnist for *Bloomberg Opinion*.

Mr. Schenker attends OPEC and Fed events, and he has given keynotes for private companies, public corporations, industry groups, and the U.S. Federal Reserve. He has advised NATO and the U.S. government on the future of work, blockchain, Bitcoin, cryptocurrency, quantum computing, data analysis, forecasting, and fake news. Mr. Schenker has written 22 books. Eleven have been #1 Best Sellers, including: *Jobs for Robots*, *Quantum: Computing Nouveau*, *Commodity Prices 101*, *Recession-Proof*, *Futureproof Supply Chain*, *Electing Recession*, *The Future of Finance is Now*, *The Future of Energy*, *The Dumpster Fire Election*, and *The Robot and Automation Almanac* for 2018 and 2020. Mr. Schenker also wrote *The Promise of Blockchain*, *Futureproof Supply Chain*, *The Fog of Data*, *Robot-Proof Yourself*, *Financial Risk Management Fundamentals*, *Midterm Economics*, *Spikes: Growth Hacking Leadership*, *Reading the Economic Tea Leaves*, and *Be the Shredder, Not the Shred*. Mr. Schenker was featured as one of the world's foremost futurists in the book *After Shock*.

Mr. Schenker advises executives, industry groups, institutional investors, and central banks as the President of Prestige Economics. He also founded The Futurist Institute in October 2016, for which he created a rigorous course of study that includes *The Future of Work*, *The Future of Transportation*, *The Future of Data*, *The Future of Finance*, *Futurist Fundamentals*, *The Future of Energy*, *The Future of Leadership*, *The Future of Healthcare, and The Future of Quantum Computing*. Mr. Schenker is also an instructor for LinkedIn Learning courses on *Corporate Finance Risk Management*, *Audit and Due Diligence*, *Recession-Proof Strategies*, and a weekly *Economic Indicator* series. He has three forthcoming LinkedIn Learning courses on business and finance leadership.

Mr. Schenker holds a Master's in Applied Economics from UNC Greensboro, a Master's in Negotiation, Conflict Resolution, and Peacebuilding from CSU Dominguez Hills, a Master's in Germanic Languages and Literature from UNC Chapel Hill, and a Bachelor's in History and German from The University of Virginia. He also holds a Certificate in FinTech from MIT, a Certificate in Supply Chain Management from MIT, a Certificate in Professional Development from UNC, a Certificate in Negotiation from Harvard Law School, a Certificate in Cybersecurity from Carnegie Mellon, and a Professional Certificate in Strategic Foresight from the University of Houston. Mr. Schenker holds the designations CMT® (Chartered Market Technician), ERP® (Energy Risk Professional), and CFP® (Certified Financial Planner). He is also a Certified Futurist and Long-Term Analyst™ and holds the FLTA™ designation.

Before founding Prestige Economics, Mr. Schenker worked as a Risk Specialist at McKinsey and Company, where he provided content direction to trading, risk, and commodity project teams on six continents. Prior to McKinsey, Mr. Schenker was the Chief Energy and Commodity Economist at Wachovia, which is now Wells Fargo. Based in Austin, Mr. Schenker is one of only 100 CEOs on the Texas Business Leadership Council, a non-partisan organization that advises Texas elected leadership at the state and federal level. Mr. Schenker is a Governance Fellow of the National Association of Corporate Directors. He also sits on multiple boards and is the VP of Finance on the Executive Committee of The Texas Lyceum, the preeminent non-partisan leadership group in Texas.

FI THE FUTURIST INSTITUTE

The Futurist Institute was founded in 2016 to help analysts, executives, and professionals incorporate new and emerging technology risk into their strategic planning. The Futurist Institute confers the Futurist and Long-Term Analyst™ (FLTA) designation and helps analysts become Certified Futurists™. Our courses have been approved for continuing education hours by the Certified Financial Planner Board of Standards (CFP Board), Global Association of Risk Professionals (GARP), and National Association of Certified Valuators and Analysts (NACVA).

Current Courses

The Future of Work
The Future of Data
The Future of Energy
The Future of Finance
The Future of Healthcare
The Future of Leadership
The Future of Transportation
Futurist Fundamentals
Quantum Computing

Visit The Futurist Institute:

www.futuristinstitute.org

PUBLISHER

Prestige Professional Publishing was founded in 2011 to produce insightful and timely professional reference books. We are registered with the Library of Congress.

Published Titles

Be the Shredder, Not the Shred
Commodity Prices 101
Electing Recession
Financial Risk Management Fundamentals
Futureproof Supply Chain
A Gentle Introduction to Audit and Due Diligence
Jobs for Robots
Midterm Economics
Quantum: Computing Nouveau
Reading the Economic Tea Leaves
Robot-Proof Yourself
Spikes: Growth Hacking Leadership
The Dumpster Fire Election
The Fog of Data
The Future After COVID
The Future of Energy
The Future of Finance is Now
The Promise of Blockchain
The Robot and Automation Almanac — 2018
The Robot and Automation Almanac — 2019
The Robot and Automation Almanac — 2020

PUBLISHER

Future Titles

Content Monster
Disruption Warfare
The Future of Agriculture
The Future of Healthcare
The Future of Travel and Leisure

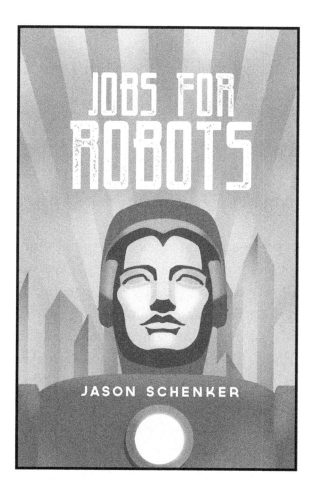

Jobs for Robots provides an in-depth look at the future of automation and robots, with a focus on the opportunities as well as the risks ahead. Job creation in coming years will be extremely strong for the kind of workers that do not require payroll taxes, healthcare, or vacation: robots. *Jobs for Robots* was published in February 2017. This book has been a #1 Best Seller on Amazon.

DISCLAIMER

FROM THE AUTHOR

The following disclaimer applies to any content in this book:

This book is commentary intended for general information use only and is not investment advice. Jason Schenker does not make recommendations on any specific or general investments, investment types, asset classes, non-regulated markets, specific equities, bonds, or other investment vehicles. Jason Schenker does not guarantee the completeness or accuracy of analyses and statements in this book, nor does Jason Schenker assume any liability for any losses that may result from the reliance by any person or entity on this information. Opinions, forecasts, and information are subject to change without notice. This book does not represent a solicitation or offer of financial or advisory services or products; this book is only market commentary intended and written for general information use only. This book does not constitute investment advice. All links were correct and active at the time this book was published.

DISCLAIMER

FROM THE PUBLISHER

The following disclaimer applies to any content in this book:

This book is commentary intended for general information use only and is not investment advice. Prestige Professional Publishing, LLC does not make recommendations on any specific or general investments, investment types, asset classes, non-regulated markets, specific equities, bonds, or other investment vehicles. Prestige Professional Publishing, LLC does not guarantee the completeness or accuracy of analyses and statements in this book, nor does Prestige Professional Publishing, LLC assume any liability for any losses that may result from the reliance by any person or entity on this information. Opinions, forecasts, and information are subject to change without notice. This book does not represent a solicitation or offer of financial or advisory services or products; this book is only market commentary intended and written for general information use only. This book does not constitute investment advice. All links were correct and active at the time this book was published.

Prestige Professional Publishing, LLC

4412 City Park Road #4

Austin, Texas 78730

www.prestigeprofessionalpublishing.com

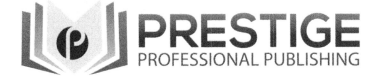

ISBN: 978-1-946197-48-1 *Paperback*
978-1-946197-51-1 *Ebook*